**MIKOLA BOGOMOLOV**
**INNA PARFILO**

# BLOOD GLUCOSE MEASURING DEVICE WITH INTEGRATED PATCH ANTENNA

MIKOLA BOGOMOLOV

INNA PARFILO

# BLOOD GLUCOSE MEASURING DEVICE WITH INTEGRATED PATCH ANTENNA

## MEASURING GLUCOSE IN THE BLOOD

ScienciaScripts

**Imprint**

Any brand names and product names mentioned in this book are subject to trademark, brand or patent protection and are trademarks or registered trademarks of their respective holders. The use of brand names, product names, common names, trade names, product descriptions etc. even without a particular marking in this work is in no way to be construed to mean that such names may be regarded as unrestricted in respect of trademark and brand protection legislation and could thus be used by anyone.

Cover image: www.ingimage.com

This book is a translation from the original published under ISBN 978-620-7-65393-5.

Publisher:
Sciencia Scripts
is a trademark of
Dodo Books Indian Ocean Ltd. and OmniScriptum S.R.L publishing group

120 High Road, East Finchley, London, N2 9ED, United Kingdom
Str. Armeneasca 28/1, office 1, Chisinau MD-2012, Republic of Moldova, Europe
Printed at: see last page
**ISBN: 978-620-7-90882-0**

# BOGOMOLOV M.F., PARFILO I.O.

## ABSTRACT

**Relevance of the topic:** Most rapid glucose testing methods require a finger prick, which is quite inconvenient for people with diabetes. Because of this, much research has focused on finding an alternative, namely a painless, minimally invasive method for glucose monitoring.

**Objective:** Non-invasive blood glucose measurement using a patch antenna.

To achieve this goal, the following tasks have been set:

1. Conduct a patent search for glucometers and a literature search for non-invasive methods of blood glucose monitoring.

2. Analyze the use of antennas as a method of measuring blood glucose and provide formulas for calculating parameters and specifications.

3. Construct a block diagram of a useful model of a device for measuring blood glucose with an integrated patch antenna.

4. Develop a model of the patch antenna and analyze its compliance with the planned technical characteristics.

5. Create a model of the finger phantom and measure the parameter S11 for different glucose concentrations in the finger phantom at different positions around the antenna.

**Keywords:** glucose, glucometer, patch antenna, dielectric constant, measurement.

# TABLE OF CONTENTS

# INTRODUCTION

Diabetes mellitus (DM) is a group of metabolic disorders characterized by hyperglycemia in the absence of treatment. The main characteristic of diabetes is impaired insulin secretion, its action, or both [1].

Today, the number of people with diabetes is approximately 537 million, and according to the WHO report, the prevalence of diabetes among people over 18 is 8.5%. In Ukraine, more than 1.2 million cases are officially registered, although studies show that for every registered case, there are 2-3 undiagnosed cases, which suggests that the real number may reach 3.4-4 million [2].

One of the most pressing issues in modern endocrinology is the possibility of early diagnosis of diabetes and treatment of its complications. Patients with diabetes should constantly monitor their blood glucose levels and, accordingly, inject the correct dose of insulin into the body. Rapid glucose testing is performed using glucose meters. The problem is that most glucometers require a finger prick, which is quite inconvenient for many people. Because of this, many studies have focused on finding an alternative, namely painless minimally invasive glucose monitoring [3].

Objective: Non-invasive blood glucose measurement using a patch antenna.

Objectives:

1. Conduct a patent search for glucometers and a literature search for non-invasive methods of blood glucose monitoring.

2. Analyze the use of antennas as a method of measuring blood glucose and provide formulas for calculating parameters and specifications.

3. Build a block diagram of a useful model of a device for measuring blood glucose with an integrated patch antenna.

4. Develop a model of the patch antenna and analyze its compliance with the planned technical characteristics.

5. Create a model of the finger phantom and measure the parameter S11 for different glucose concentrations in the finger phantom.

# SECTION I
# LITERATURE ANALYSIS
## 1.1 Definition and classification of diabetes mellitus

Diabetes mellitus (DM) is a group of metabolic disorders characterized by hyperglycemia in the absence of treatment. The main characteristic of diabetes is impaired insulin secretion, its action, or both [1].

It has been reported that up to 3 million people die every year due to this disease, or one death every 10 seconds [4]. Today, the number of people with diabetes is approximately 450 million, and according to the World Health Organization, the prevalence of diabetes among people over 18 is 8.5%. In Ukraine, more than 1.2 million cases are officially registered, although studies show that for every registered case there are 2-3 undiagnosed cases, which suggests that the real number may reach 3.4-4 million [2].

Consider the main types of diabetes mellitus (Fig. 1.1) [5]. The most common are types 1 and 2.

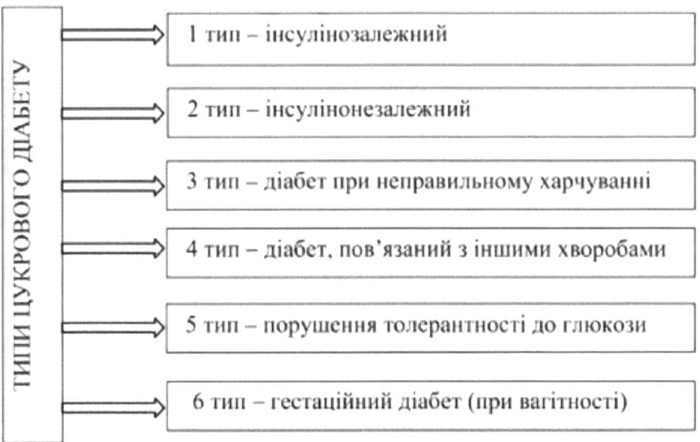


Figure 1.1 - Types of diabetes mellitus

Type 1 diabetes (or insulin-dependent type) is characterized by insufficient or complete cessation of insulin synthesis in the body and the need for injections to maintain its level in the blood [6]. This is due to changes in the pancreatic cells *(β-cells)* that produce insulin, which can be caused by environmental factors, viral infections, and genetic mechanisms [5].

Type 2 diabetes (insulin-independent type) is characterized by the fact that the body produces enough insulin, but it is not absorbed by the body's cells due to resistance. Most often, this form occurs at the age of 50-70 and is the most common [6]. This type occurs gradually and is often diagnosed incidentally during an examination [5].

The clinical characteristics of type 1, type 2 diabetes and gestational diabetes are given in (Table 1.1) [2].

Table 1.1 - Clinical characteristics of different types of diabetes mellitus

| Symptoms | Diabetes mellitus | | |
|---|---|---|---|
| | Type 1 | Type 2 | gestational |
| A sharp start | + | - | - |
| Excessive body weight | - | + | -\+ |
| Steady course | - | + | + |
| Ketoacidosis | + | - | - |
| Reducing the level of insulin in the blood | + | - | + |
| Increased levels of C-peptide | - | + | - |
| Pancreatic P-cell antibodies | + | - | + |
| Association with HLA alleles | + | - | + |
| The need for exogenous insulin | + | - | + |
| Late complications: microangiopathies | + | - | + |

Gestational diabetes occurs for the first time in women during pregnancy. It is caused by the physiological development of insulin resistance due to excessive production of placental hormones, physiological insulin antagonists. The disease resolves on its own [7].


## 1.1.1 Type 1 diabetes mellitus


Type 1 diabetes is an autoimmune disease characterized by the gradual destruction of pancreatic *β-cells,* which leads to a lack of insulin. The causes of type 1 diabetes can be described as follows:

- the presence of histocompatibility antigens (*HLA-B8, B16, B15, B35, DR3, DR4, DR3/DR4, DQA-Arg52+/DQB-Asp57,* etc;)

- genetic determination, namely the sensitivity of *β-cells* to antigens or the ability to antiviral immunity;

- the presence of genes responsible for insulin synthesis (chromosome 11) or those related to immunoglobulins and blood groups;

- environmental exposure (triggers are viruses, chemicals, toxins, *β-tropic* viruses, cytotoxic substances) with the appearance of antigens [2].

Symptoms of type 1 diabetes can be divided into two groups:

- caused by decompensation of the disease;

- caused by the presence of diabetic angiopathy, neuropathy and other complications of the disease.

Compensation of diabetes mellitus is the maintenance of the main indicators of carbohydrate, fat, protein and electrolyte metabolism at a level close to the norm, which ensures a satisfactory condition of the patient and his or her performance. Therefore, in turn, the symptoms of decompensation include: polydipsia (thirst), polyuria (increased urine production), nocturia (frequent need to urinate at night), dry mouth, itchy skin, rapid weight loss, weakness, and weight loss [8].

This type of diabetes usually develops in children and people under 40 years of age. The number of people with this type is 10-13% of the total number of patients with diabetes [6].

## 1.1.2 Type 2 diabetes mellitus

According to research, this disease has a polygenic inheritance. External factors that contribute to the development of the disease include overeating and physical inactivity, which in turn lead to obesity. Obesity is observed in almost 80% of patients with type 2 diabetes.

The greatest risk of development is with:

- elderly people;

- identical twins, one of whom has diabetes;

- women who have given birth to a child weighing 4.5 kg or more;

- persons with one or both parents suffering from diabetes;

- women with children with developmental disabilities;

- persons with renal and nutritional glucosuria, which occurs episodically in stressful situations;

- persons suffering from hypertension, atherosclerosis, obesity, hyperuricemia, gout;

- patients with diseases of the biliary tract and liver, pancreas, chronic urinary tract infections, CKD and respiratory system;

- patients with manifestations of metabolic syndrome (IR, hypertension, hyperinsulinemia, hyperuricemia, increased platelet aggregation, microalbuminuria);

- patients with neuropathies of unclear etiology.

Type 2 diabetes is characterized by a slow development of the disease, especially in the elderly. Complaints caused by diabetes decompensation may be episodic. Thirst and polyuria increase in the evening and after meals. However, in the setting of infection, intoxication, and trauma, type 2 diabetes can manifest itself quite acutely [9].

## 1.2 Analysis of existing glucose meters available on the Ukrainian market

One of the most pressing issues in modern endocrinology is the possibility of early diagnosis of diabetes and treatment of its complications. Patients with diabetes must constantly monitor their metabolic state (determining blood glucose levels) and, accordingly, administer the correct dose of insulin to the body. Rapid glucose testing is performed using glucose meters.

At present, there are more than 200 commercial insulin products in the world, each with its own clinical and pharmacological characteristics and different duration of action. About 85% of all insulin products are manufactured by these companies: Novo Nordisk (Denmark), Bioton (Poland), Lilly France (France), Sanofi-Aventis (Germany). In Ukraine, industrial production of insulin began in 1999 [10].

Glucometers are divided into photometric and electrochemical according to the principle of operation. Photometric glucometers determine the concentration of glucose by changing the color of the reagent, which occurs as a result of the reaction of glucose with special substances on the test strip [11]. The main enzymes of the test strips are glucose oxidase and glucose dehydrogenase. The color change is recorded using a spectrometer [10]. Electrochemical glucometers determine the level of glucose by measuring the current that occurs when glucose and reagents applied to the test strip interact [11].

### 1.2.1. FreeStyle Libre

*Freestyle Libre* uses subcutaneous, wire-based technology to measure glucose levels in interstitial fluid. This glucose meter belongs to the minimally invasive category, as the puncture is made using a thin thread that is only advanced in the upper layers of the skin. The sensor stays on the body for up to 14 days [10].

Figure 1.2 shows the appearance of the glucometer:

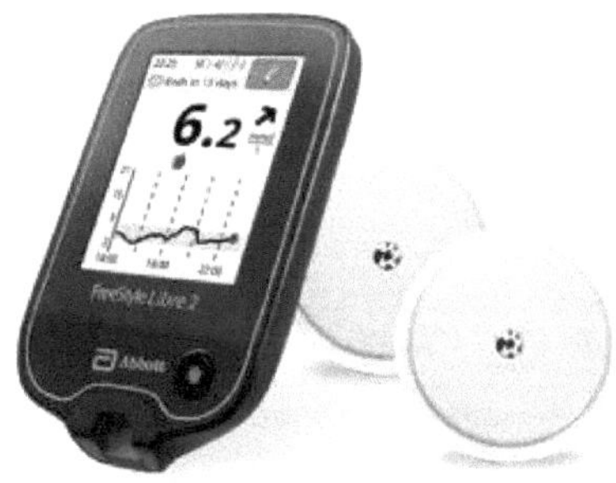

Figure 1.2 - Exterior of the *Freestyle Libre* glucose meter

*The Freestyle Libre* sensor automatically measures glucose levels every minute, and the results are stored in 15-minute intervals. The reader is held next to the sensor whenever you want to take a glucose reading. It displays glucose information for the last 8 hours, including the current glucose level and a trend graph [12]. Technical characteristics are given in (Table 1.2) [13]:

Table 1.2 - Technical characteristics of *Freestyle Libre*

| Method of measuring glucose levels | Electrochemical |
|---|---|
| Sensor size | Height 5 mm, diameter 35 mm |
| The range of blood glucose determination | 20 - 500 mg/dL |

| Weight of the sensor | 5 г |
| --- | --- |
| Maximum number of days of detector operation | 14 days |

Advantages of the *Freestyle Libre* sensor:

- the procedure for measuring glucose levels is absolutely painless;

- the sensor does not interfere with or cause discomfort;

- lack of a calibration procedure;

- *Freestyle Libre* is completely waterproof [13].

Disadvantages of the *Freestyle Libre* sensor:

- *the FreeStyle Libre* sensor is located in tissues, not in blood. This means that the data may lag by 15-20 minutes [10];

- the device shows inaccuracies at lower glucose levels. In 40% of the cases where the device showed that the patient's glucose level was <60 mg/dL, the actual glucose level was within the normal range (81-160 mg/dL) [12].

## 1.2.2 Accu - Chek Active

The blood glucose monitoring system consists of a glucose meter and test strips. The *Accu-Chek Active* glucose meter is designed to quantify glucose levels in fresh capillary blood and can only be used in conjunction with *Accu-Chek Active* test strips [14].

Figure 1.3 shows the appearance of the glucometer:

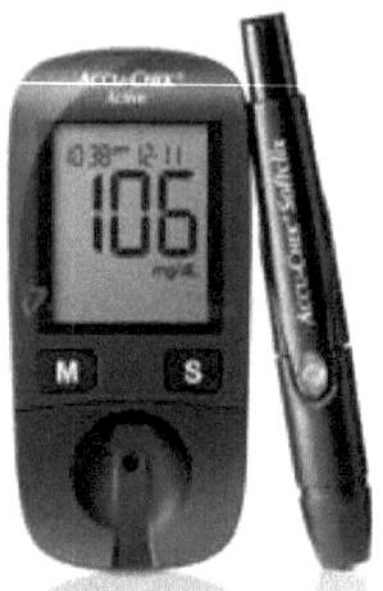

Figure 1.3 - Exterior of the *Accu-Chek Active* glucose meter

Technical characteristics are given in (Table 1.3) [15]:

Table 1.3 - Technical characteristics of *Accu-Chek Active*

| Method of measuring glucose levels | photometric |
|---|---|
| Dimensions | 97.8 x 46.8 x 19.1 mm |
| The range of blood glucose determination | 0.6 - 33.3 mmol/l |
| Weight | 50 g with battery |
| Calibration | Whole blood |
| Memory. | 500 results |
| Measurement time | 5 seconds |
| The volume of a drop of blood | 1-2 µl |

Advantages of the *Accu-Chek Active* glucose meter:

- easy to use. Large display, getting the result without pressing buttons;

- no need for coding;

- the ability to transfer data to a PC;

- the glucose meter remembers the last 500 tests.

Disadvantages of the *Accu-Chek Active* glucose meter:

- a finger puncture is necessary;

- there may be small errors in glucose measurement [15].

## 1.2.3 One Touch Select Simple

Technical specifications are given in (Table 1.4):

Table 1.4 - Technical specifications of *One Touch Select Simple*

| Method of measuring glucose levels | electrochemical |
|---|---|
| Dimensions | 86 x 51 x 16 mm |
| The range of blood glucose determination | 1.1 - 33.3 mmol / l |
| Weight | 43 g with battery |
| Calibration | Whole blood |
| Measurement time | 5 seconds |
| The volume of a drop of blood | 0.5 µl |

Figure 1.4 shows the appearance of the glucometer:

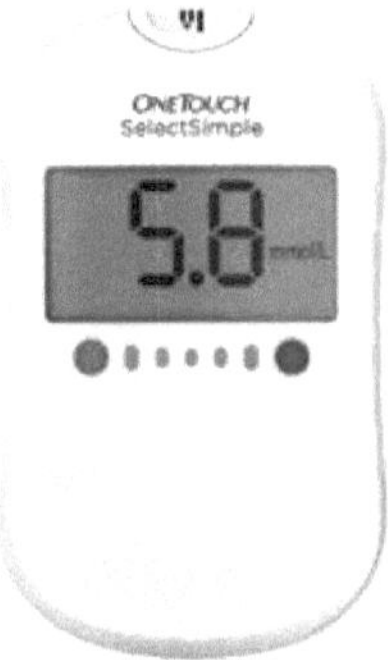


Figure 1.4 - Exterior of the *One Touch Select* Simple glucose meter

Advantages of the *One Touch Select Simple* glucose meter:

- *The One Touch Select Simple* glucose meter is easy to use;

- The device alerts you if the measurement result is low [20-69 mg/dL (1.1-3.8 mmol/L)], high [180-239 mg/dL (9.9-13.2 mmol/L)], or very high [240-600 mg/dL (13.3-33.1 mmol/L)] glucose [16].

Disadvantages of the *One Touch Select Simple* glucose meter:

- the package contains only ten test strips. For further use, test strips must be purchased separately;

- data is not saved. The glucose meter does not provide the ability to synchronize its readings with a digital device;

- The battery lasts for one month [17].

## 1.2.4 Longevita Smart

*The Longevita Smart* glucose meter has the function of displaying the analysis result, time and date of the glucose measurement on the display. Figure 1.5 shows the appearance of *Longevita Smart*:

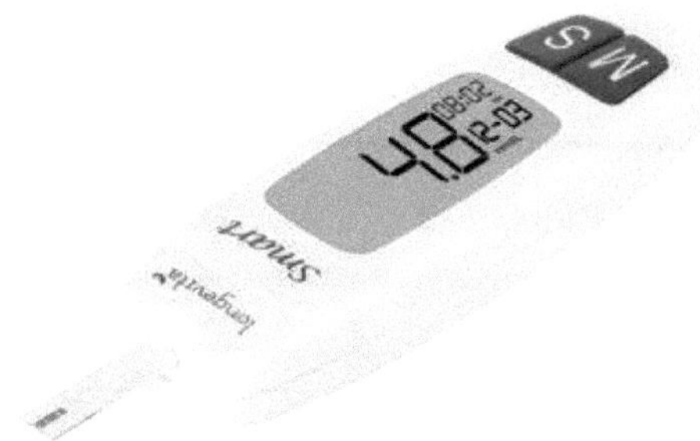

Figure 5 - appearance of the *Longevita Smart* glucose meter

The technical characteristics of this are given in (Table 1.5) [18]:

Table 1.5 - Technical characteristics of *Longevita Smart*

| Method of measuring glucose levels | Electrochemical |
|---|---|
| Dimensions | 150x115x45mm |
| The range of blood glucose determination | 1.1 - 33.3 mmol / l |
| Weight | 50 г |
| Calibration | Whole blood |
| Memory. | 360 measurements |
| Measurement time | 5 sec |
| The volume of a drop of blood | 1 μl |

## 1.2.5 Comparison of glucose meter characteristics

A comparison of the above glucose meters is given in (Table 1.6). From this table, it can be determined that the widest range of glucose determination is provided by the *Accu-Chek Active* glucose meter, *and the smallest - by the Freestyle Libre*. This can be explained by the fact that, unlike other glucometers, *Freestyle Libre is minimally* invasive. At the same time, it is the smallest in size and does not require finger pricking. The *One Touch Select Simple* and *Longevita Smart* glucometers are very similar to each other, except for size.

Table 1.6 - Comparison of glucose meters characteristics

| Name of the glucose meter | Method of measuring glucose levels | Dimensions | Calibration | Measurement time | The range of blood glucose determination |
|---|---|---|---|---|---|
| Freestyle Libre | Electrochemical | Height 5 mm, diameter 35 mm | - | automatically measures glucose levels every minute | 20 - 500 mg/dL (1.11 - 27.78 mmol/L) |
| Accu-Chek Active | photometric | 97.8 x 46.8 x 19.1 mm | Whole blood | 5 sec | 0.6 - 33.3 mmol / 1 |
| One Touch Select Simple | Electrochemical | 86 x 51 x 16 mm | Whole blood | 5 sec | 1.1 - 33.3 mmol / 1 |
| Longevita Smart | Electrochemical | 150x115x4.5mm | Whole blood | 5 sec | 1.1 - 33.3 mmol / 1 |

Conclusions to Section I

In this section, we have discussed the types of glucometers and their classification. Photometric glucose meters use a spectrometer to measure the change in color of the reagent on the test strip after it reacts with glucose, while electrochemical glucose meters measure the current that occurs when glucose reacts with the reagents on the test strip.

The characteristics of the glucometers were also compared, namely: measurement method, size, calibration, measurement time, and blood glucose range.

# NON-INVASIVE METHODS OF BLOOD GLUCOSE MONITORING

## 2.1 Description and analysis of the most studied non-invasive methods of blood glucose monitoring

Basically, methods for measuring blood glucose levels are divided into invasive, minimally invasive, and non-invasive. Invasive methods require blood sampling from patients with diabetes. The amount of blood depends on the monitoring method. For example, clinical laboratory tests require 1-3 ml of blood sample to analyze glucose levels, with the hexokinase method used as a reference standard for diagnosing diabetes [19].

Electromagnetic and optical methods use non-ionizing waves, and each frequency range and wavelength has its advantages and disadvantages. In optical methods, the terahertz (THz) range is able to penetrate the skin superficially, interacting mainly with the epidermis. Also, the penetration of THz waves depends on the light intensity, tissue properties, and wavelength.

Four interactions can occur when electromagnetic waves pass through biological tissue: scattering, reflection, absorption, and transmission. When the waves are directed to the surface of the tissue and reflected from it, this is called reflection. The characteristics and intensity of the reflected waves are analyzed in this method. In scattering methods, the wave is directed into the tissue, where it interacts with the tissue, scatters, and exits at a specific angle. In absorption, tissues absorb specific wavelengths of electromagnetic waves. The amount of light absorbed can provide the necessary information about the concentration of substances in the tissue.

Thus, by analyzing the behavior of electromagnetic waves in the tissue, it is possible to collect information about the concentration of glucose in the tissue [20].

## 2.1.1 Near-infrared spectroscopy

Spectroscopy is a branch of physics that studies the laws of interaction of electromagnetic radiation (light) with a chemical substance. Such interactions can be accompanied by absorption, emission or scattering of electromagnetic radiation.

Vibrations of atoms in a molecule, which are accompanied by a change in dipole moment (charge shift), have their own resonant absorption frequencies in the infrared region (IR). The infrared region of electromagnetic radiation is divided into the near-infrared (wavelength 700 nm - 2.5 μm), the infrared itself (2.5-25 μm) and the far infrared (25-600 μm) regions. The infrared spectra of each molecule are absolutely specific, so they can be considered as a kind of "fingerprints" of molecules [21, p. 115].

The reflection and absorption of light of a certain wavelength causes corresponding molecular vibrations in glucose that can be observed in its spectra. The molecular vibrations that exist in the general near-infrared region are called overtones.

The structure of a glucose molecule is shown in (Figure 2.1). In the long-wavelength near-infrared region (700-1300 nm), vibrations between *OH* and *CH* were detected, which are called the first overtone. Thus, the glucose molecule can be detected [22].

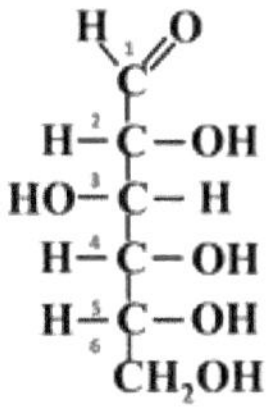

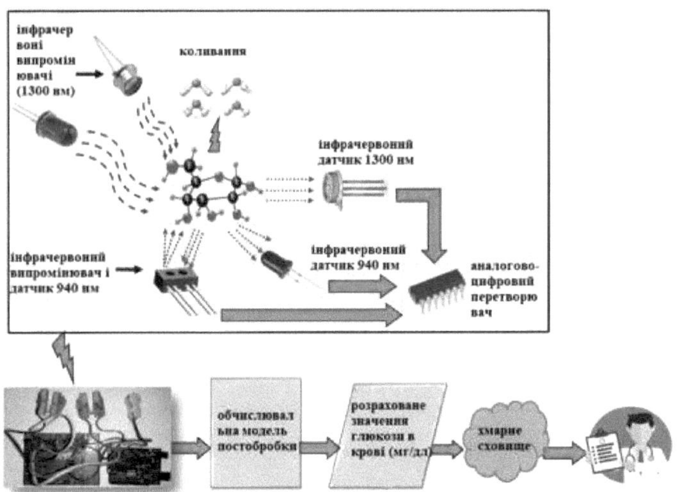

Figure 2.1 - Atomic structure of a glucose molecule

For example, the *iGLU* 1.0 glucose meter (Figure 2.2) uses the concept of short-wave *NIR spectroscopy* with two different wavelengths (940 and 1300 nm).



Figure 2.2 - Conceptual overview of *iGLU* 1.0

This device is implemented using three channels and uses the *IoMT* platform for data storage and remote monitoring.

Three channels, each with its own emitter and detector, are used to collect data. The data is processed by a 16-bit analog-to-digital converter with a sampling rate of 128 samples per second. Regression analysis methods are used to calibrate and verify the data.

The data stored in the cloud can be used and monitored by patients and doctors. It is an inexpensive device with an accuracy of more than 90%, but it does not provide real-time results [23].

The main disadvantage of the long-wave near-infrared region is the shallow penetration of light compared to the short-wave near-infrared region (1300 - 2500 nm). At the same time, the short wave has a rather weak absorption of the glucose molecule compared to the long wave. Thus, it is better to use short-wave near-infrared spectroscopy in research [22].

### 2.1.2 Raman spectroscopy

Raman spectroscopy is a non-destructive chemical analysis technique that provides detailed information about chemical structure, polymorphism, phases, molecular interactions, and crystallinity.

Raman analysis is a light scattering technique whereby a molecule scatters light incident from a high-intensity laser. Most of the scattered light has the same wavelength as the laser source and does not carry any useful information - this is called Rayleigh scattering. However, a small amount of light (typically 0.0000001%) is scattered by different wavelengths that depend on the chemical structure of the molecule - this is the so-called Raman scattering [24].

Since the depth of penetration of laser light is very small (it is only 200 microns), the laser cannot reach the dermis, where there are microvessels. Therefore, in a Raman test for blood glucose, scientists usually only obtain the Raman spectrum of the stratum corneum and epidermis [25].

As shown in (Figure 2.3), the simplest structure of a Raman spectrometer consists of a lens that captures part of the scattered radiation and directs it to a filter that transmits only Raman scattered light. A computer processes the signal and provides the corresponding Raman shift [26].

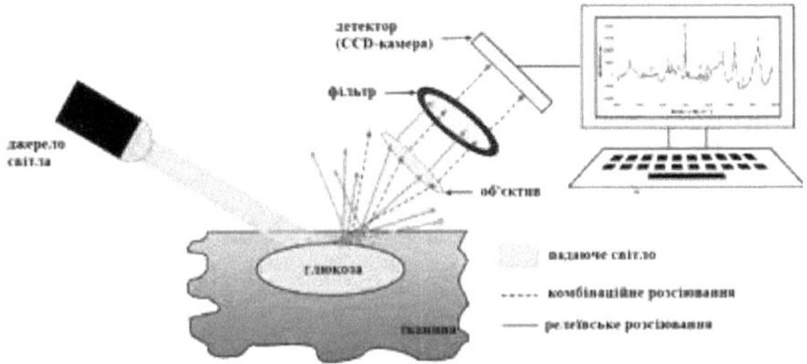


Figure 2.3 - Schematic representation of the device for Raman spectroscopy

### 2.1.3 Polarimetry

Polarimetry is an optical analysis technique that measures the optical rotational dispersion caused by an optically active molecule. Glucose exhibits various forms of isomerism, in particular, it forms two optical chiral isomers, *D-glucose* and *L-glucose*. The enantiomers are mirror images of each other, so *D-glucose* will rotate the plane of polarized light clockwise, while *L-glucose* will rotate the plane counterclockwise.

*D-glucose is* naturally occurring, while *L-glucose has* been produced only synthetically. The principle of polarimetry is to determine the concentration of glucose by the angle at which polarized light is returned [27].

Figure 2.4 shows a schematic of a polarimeter and its components: light source, sample, polarization analyzer, linear polarizer, and photodetector.

Unpolarized light is characterized as an electric field that oscillates in many planes relative to the propagation axis.

An ideal linear polarizer can filter a light source in such a way that the electric field inside the light source oscillates in only one plane, in this case perpendicular to the sample surface. Thus, the polarized light passes through the sample, and the glucose molecules contained in it cause the angle of the electric field to rotate from its original angle. The polarizer is also used as a polarization analyzer to determine the plane of the polarized light after it passes through the sample. When the polarization axis in the analyzer coincides with the angle of rotation ($\theta$) of the electric field, the maximum light intensity will be detected by the photodetector [28].

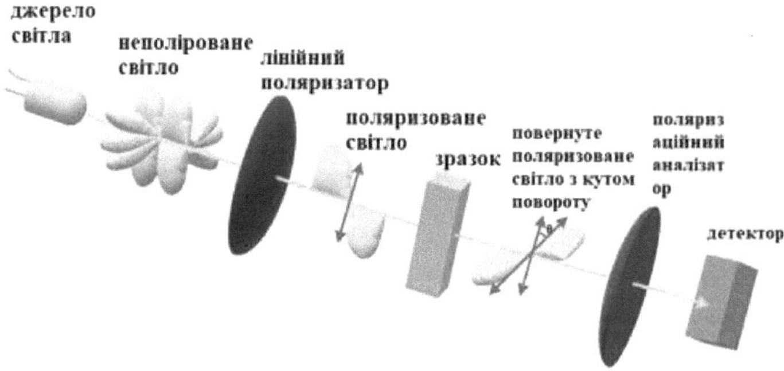


Figure 2.4 - Simplified diagram of a polarimeter

However, the skin is not very well suited for polarimetry due to the high level of scattering that causes depolarization. For this reason, almost all polarimetry studies have focused on the aqueous humor of the eye [20]. Light can pass almost tangentially through the aqueous humor or be reflected off the retina, and most studies have used one of these approaches (Figure 2.5). Complications arise because the glucose level in the aqueous humor is different from that in the blood: studies show that the glucose level in the aqueous humor is 70% of that in the blood. There is also a time delay, which in rabbits is about 5 minutes, and modeling suggests that in humans it can be up to 7 minutes.

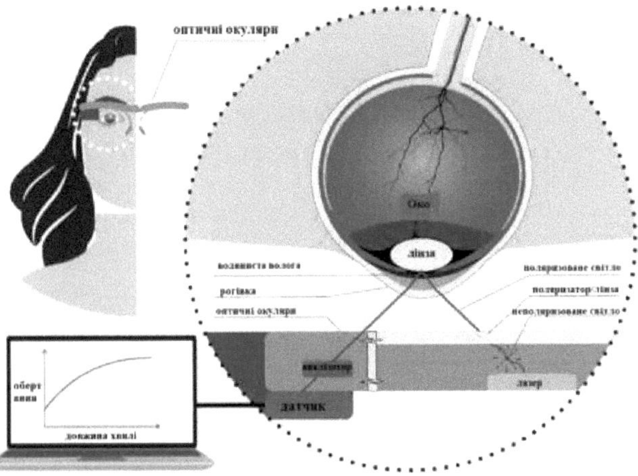


Figure 2.5 - Polarimetry method for determining glucose in the human eye

From a practical point of view, there are safety issues when using strong light sources [27].

## 2.1.4 Mid-infrared spectroscopy

As with near-infrared spectroscopy, mid-infrared (*MIR)* spectroscopy is used to obtain numerical information about a sample based on absorption spectra. This spectroscopy uses a longer wavelength in the range of 2500-10,000 nm, and therefore there is less scattering and more absorption in the tissue, resulting in clear and sharp peaks in the glucose absorption spectra.

However, *MIR* can only penetrate the skin to a minimum depth of about 100 microns due to the absorption of water and other biological compounds (Figure 2.6). This limits the system's tuning for reflection, as it is not possible to measure transmittance.

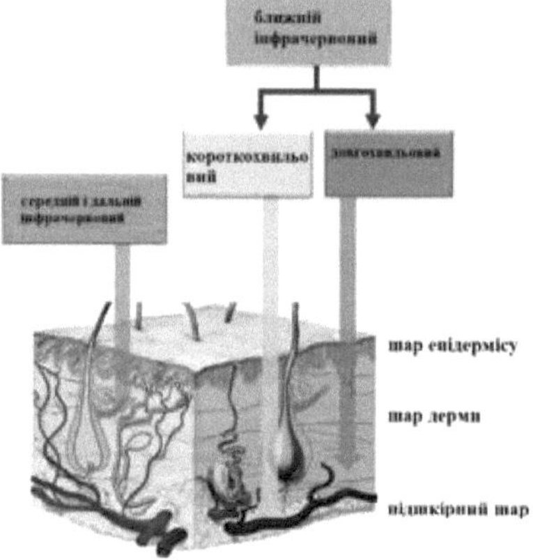


Figure 2.6 - Depth of penetration in the mid-infrared region

A method for estimating glucose concentration by measuring the absorption of *MIR light by the oral mucosa* using hollow fibers and an attenuated total reflection *(ATR) prism has* been proposed. Absorption is measured from the beam coming from the *ATR* prism, which in turn is placed between the upper and lower lips, through the hollow fiber. A simplified representation of the system is shown in (Fig. 2.7) [30]:

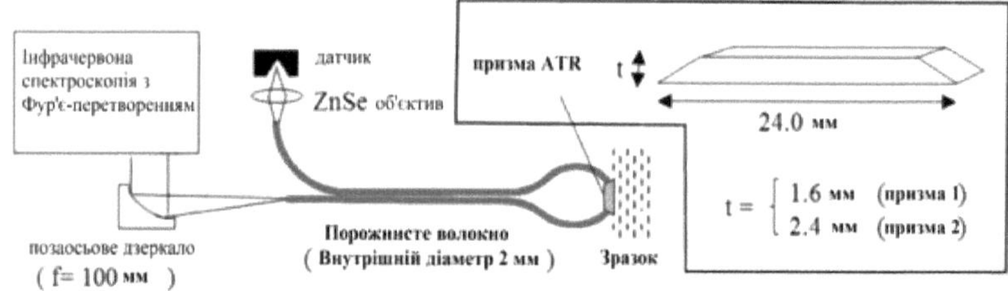


Figure 2.7 - Schematic structure of the proposed *MIR* system

## 2.2 Using antennas as a method for measuring blood glucose

## 2.2.1 Dielectric constant of blood

Dielectric constant is a measure of a material's ability to store charge. The Cole-Cole equation can be used to accurately model the dielectric behavior of biological tissues over a wide range of frequencies [30]. The dielectric constant can be determined using the following equation (2.1):

$$\varepsilon(\omega) = \varepsilon_\infty + \sum_n \frac{\Delta \varepsilon_n}{1+(j\omega\tau_n)^{(1-a_n)}} + \frac{\sigma_i}{j\omega\varepsilon_0} \tag{2.1}$$

where, $\omega$ *is the* cyclic frequency, $\varepsilon_0$ - is the dielectric constant for $\omega\tau \ll 1$, $\varepsilon_\infty$ - is the dielectric constant for $\omega\tau \gg 1$, $\alpha$ is a parameter representing the distribution of the relaxation time, $n$ is the order of the Cole-Cole model, $\sigma_i$ is the conductivity, and $\tau_m$ is the average relaxation time [32].

In people without diabetes, blood glucose levels are usually maintained between 72 mg/dL and 216 mg/dL. It has been shown that dielectric constant and conductivity decrease with increasing glucose concentration. The dielectric constant shows a slight decrease in response to an increase in blood glucose, while the conductivity shows a more pronounced decrease [31].

## 2.2.2 Microstrip antennas. Classification and characteristics

In the broadest sense, an antenna is usually a structure that has a region of transition from a directional wave to a free-space wave and vice versa. In the transmit mode, the antenna converts energy into electromagnetic waves and transmits them along a transmission line into free space. In the receive mode, the antenna receives energy in the form of electromagnetic waves from free space and then transmits it along the same transmission line.

Microstrip antennas became very popular in the 1970s and were mainly used in the space industry [33].

This type of antenna has a number of advantages over traditional antennas:

- small volume, light weight;

- low cost of production;

- mechanically durable when installed on hard surfaces.

Microstrip patch antennas also have a number of disadvantages compared to conventional antennas. Below are some of their main disadvantages:

- narrow bandwidth;

- low gain;

- extraneous radiation from feeders [34].

A simplified structure is shown in (Fig. 2.8). Any microstrip antenna consists of a radiating element, a dielectric substrate, and a metal shield [35].

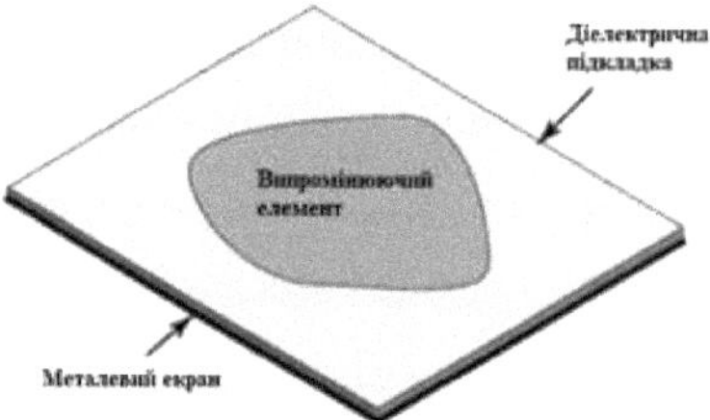


Figure 2.8 - Simplified structure of a microstrip antenna

Microstrip antennas are also often called patch antennas. The radiating element of a patch antenna can be square, circular, rectangular, thin strip (dipole), triangular, elliptical, or any other configuration. Square, rectangular, circular, and dipole radiating elements are the most common because of their ease of manufacture and low cross-polarization [36]. Figure 2.9 shows the types of radiating elements [37]:

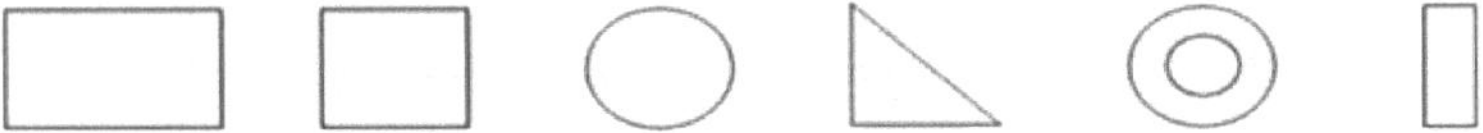

Figure 2.9 - Types of radiating elements

There are many dielectric materials that can be used for a dielectric substrate. Each dielectric has its own characteristics that affect the overall performance of the antenna. The most common dielectric materials and their properties are listed in (Table 2.1) [38]:

Table 2.1 - Dielectric materials and their characteristics

| Parameters. | FR4 | RO-4003 | RT-Duroid |
|---|---|---|---|
| Dielectric constant | 4.36 | 3.4 | 2.2 |
| Dielectric loss tangent | 0.013 | 0.002 | 0.0004 |
| water absorption (%) | <0.25 | 0.06 | 0.02 |
| Tensile strength (MPa) | 310 | 141 | 450 |
| Breakdown voltage | 55 kV | - | >60 kV |
| Density (kg/m )$^3$ | 1850 | 1790 | 2200 |

## 2.2.3 Parameters of microstrip antennas and their calculation

To determine the width of the radiating element $Wp$ of a microstrip antenna, equation (2.2) is used [39]:

$$Wp = \frac{v_0}{2 f_r} \sqrt{\frac{2}{\varepsilon_r + 1}}, (2.2)$$

where, $v_0$ - is the electromagnetic wave velocity, $f_r$ - is the resonant frequency, $\varepsilon_r$ - is the dielectric constant of the substrate.

The electric field lines of the microstrip line (Figure 2.10(a)) are shown (Figure 2.10(b)). It can be observed that most of the electric field lines are in the substrate, while some of them are in the air. In this case, the microstrip line is electrically wider compared to its physical dimensions. To take this effect into account, a new value is introduced into the antenna design - the effective permittivity $\varepsilon_{reff}$.

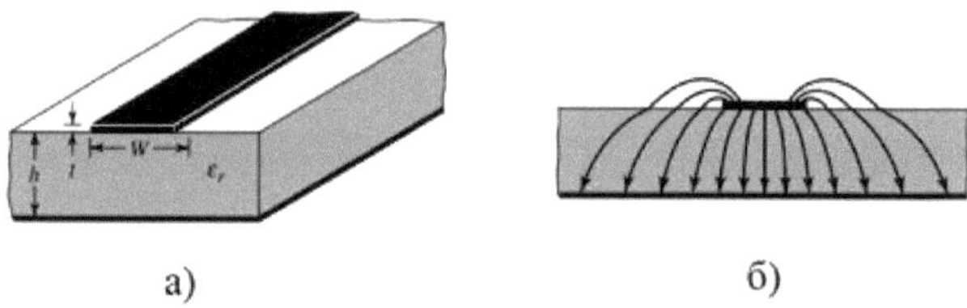


Figure 2.10 - General structure of a microstrip line a) Microstrip line; b) Electric field lines of a microstrip line

The effective permittivity is a function of frequency. At low frequencies, the effective permittivity remains virtually unchanged. As the frequency increases, its value also begins to increase and eventually approaches the value of the dielectric constant of the substrate. The initial value of the effective permittivity (at low frequencies) can be calculated using formula (2.3):

$$\varepsilon_{reff} = \frac{\varepsilon_r + 1}{2} + \frac{\varepsilon_r - 1}{2} \left[ 1 + 12 \frac{h}{Wp} \right]^{-1/2} \tag{2.3}$$

As already mentioned, the electrically radiating element of a microstrip antenna is larger than its physical dimensions. Because of this, the dimensions of the radiating element along its length were increased by a distance $\Delta L$ (at each end), which is a function of the width to height ratio (*W/h*) and the effective permittivity $\varepsilon_{reff}$ (Fig. 2.11):

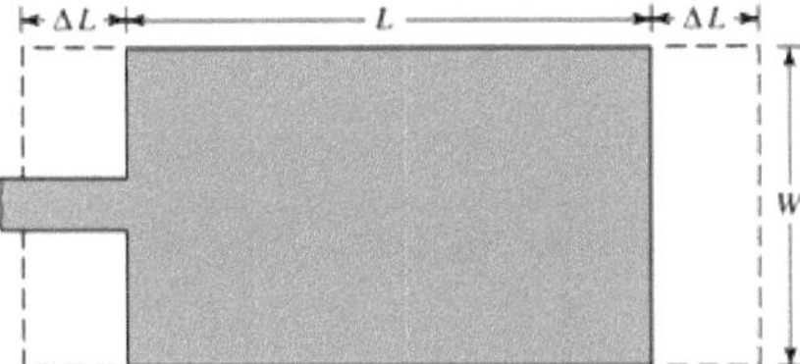

Figure 2.11 - Dimensions of the radiating element

The value of $\Delta L$ can be obtained from formula (2.4):

$$\frac{\Delta L}{h} \;=\; 0.412 \,\frac{(\varepsilon_{reff} + 0.3)\,(\frac{Wp}{h} + 0.264)}{(\varepsilon_{reff} - 0.258)\,(\frac{Wp}{h} + 0.8)} \;,\; (2.4)$$

To calculate the length of the radiating element Lp, use formula (2.5) [36]:

$$Lp \;=\; \frac{\lambda}{2} \,-\, 2\Delta L \qquad (2.5)$$

where, $\lambda$ - is the antenna radiation wavelength.

## 2.2.4 Power supply of the microstrip antenna

The patch antenna is usually powered by a coaxial probe (Fig. 2.12 (a)) or a microstrip line (Fig. 2.12 (b)):

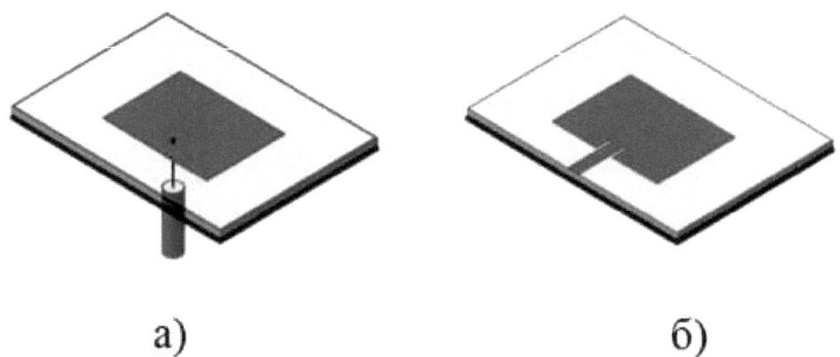



Figure 2.12 - Antenna feed types: a) Coaxial probe; b) Microstrip line

The advantages and disadvantages of these methods are shown in (Table 2.2) [35]:

Table 2.2 - Advantages and disadvantages of power supply methods

|  | Advantages. | Disadvantages |
|---|---|---|
| Coaxial probe | - easy to pick up<br>- low level of parasitic radiation | - high inductance for thick substrates<br>- soldering is required |
| Micro strip line | - easy to manufacture<br>- easy to pick up by controlling the position of the insert | parasitic radiation |

The input impedance of the patch antenna can be calculated by formula (2.6):

$$R_{in} = \frac{1}{2(G_1 \pm G_{12})} \tag{2.6}$$

where, $G_{12}$ - is the mutual conductivity, $G_1$ - is the conductivity of one slot.

The input impedance of the patch antenna will differ from the desired 50 ohm impedance. To correct this, calculate the distance to the microstrip line connection point $x_0$ from formula (2.7):

$$R_{in} = \frac{1}{2(G_1 \pm G_{12})} \left(\cos\left(\frac{\pi}{L_p} x_0\right)\right)^2 \tag{2.7}$$

The general design of the radiating element of a microstrip antenna with a microstrip feed line is shown in (Fig. 2.13) [36]:

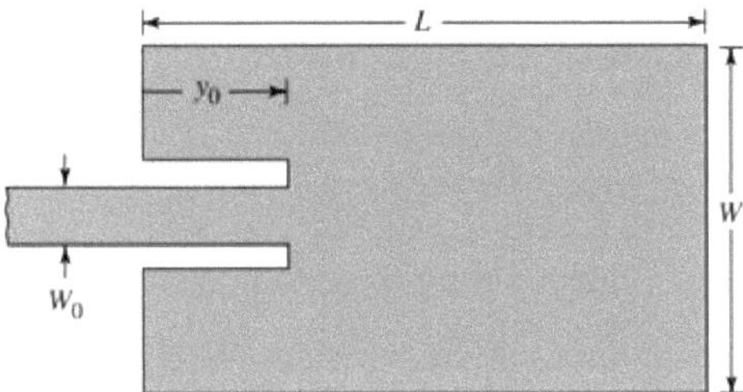


Figure 2.13 - Radiating element of a microstrip antenna with a microstrip feed line

Conclusions to Section II

In this section, we have reviewed methods of non-invasive glucose measurement, including near-infrared and mid-infrared spectroscopy, polarimetry, and Raman spectroscopy.

An overview of microstrip antennas that can be used for non-invasive blood glucose measurement was presented. This is due to the fact that the dielectric constant of blood depends on its glucose level. Therefore, we can track changes in the resonant frequency of the antenna by placing our finger on its radiating element.

# SECTION III
## DEVELOPMENT OF A USEFUL MODEL OF A DEVICE FOR MEASURING BLOOD GLUCOSE WITH AN INTEGRATED PATCH ANTENNA

### 3.1 Functional diagram of the device

The proposed scheme uses two rectangular microstrip antennas. One of them serves as a transmitting antenna (Source), and the other as a receiving antenna (Sensor). A human finger is placed between these two antennas. A signal with a resonant frequency of 2 GHz is transmitted from the Source antenna through the finger and finally received by the Sensor antenna. (Figure 3.1) illustrates the theoretical design of this system:

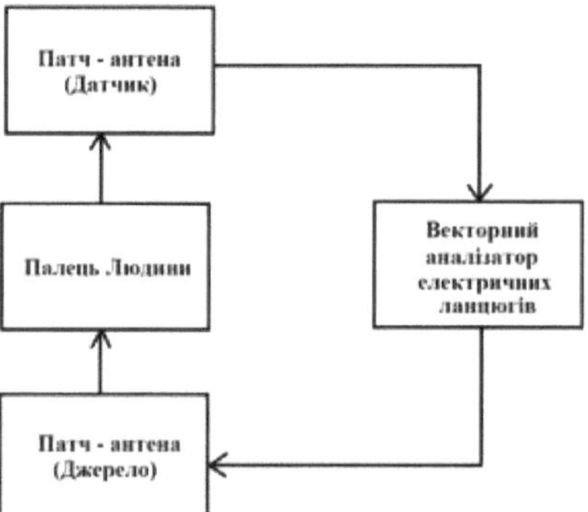


Figure 3.1 - Functional diagram of the device

A pair of microstrip patch antennas was connected to the *MS2037C* vector network analyzer (*VNA*) using an *RG 8 TZC 500 32* coaxial cable. The coaxial cables were connected to the antennas via *SMA (female) connectors*. The *VNA* was chosen to record *return loss* data - the *S11* parameter module (*reflection coefficient*). It compares the output signal from the analyzer with the signal transmitted through the test device or with the signal reflected from its input [40].

## 3.2 Modeling the finger phantom

*Ansys HFSS is a* software designed for electromagnetic *3D* modeling, design, and simulation of high-frequency electronic products. With the help of this program, designers can simulate the electromagnetic behavior of antenna structures to accurately assess potential real-life scenarios [41].

In order for the resonant frequency of the antenna to be influenced by the dielectric properties of the blood, a significant penetration depth is required. The penetration depth, in turn, depends on the operating frequency and the shape of the radiating element. As a rule, due to the inherent conductivity of biological tissues, lower frequencies achieve greater tissue penetration than higher ones [42]. The simplified structure of a human finger, which consists of a layer of skin, subcutaneous tissue, blood, bone, and nail plate, is shown in (Fig. 3.2):

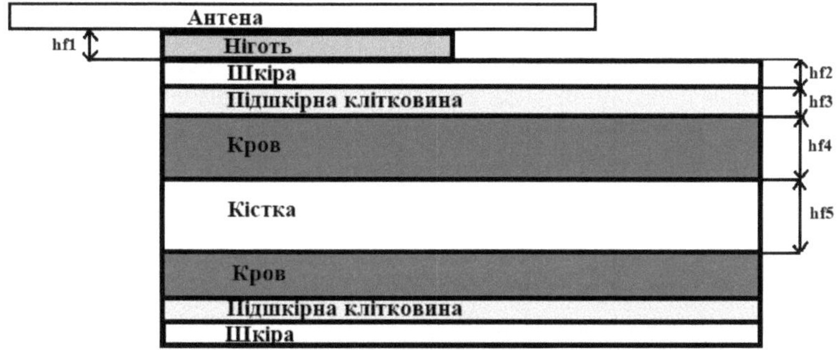


Figure 3.2 - General structure of the human finger

The penetration depths for blood and skin are shown in (Figure 3.3). It can be seen that at 2 GHz, a minimum depth of 1.5 mm is achieved for blood. Thus, the antenna should have a resonant frequency of up to 2 GHz [43].

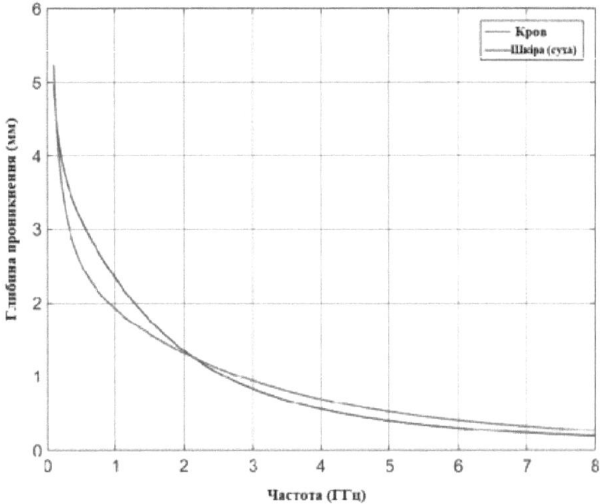



Figure 3.3 - Penetration depth for blood and skin

The dielectric constant for blood can be calculated using the Cole-Cole model. Since the dielectric constant of blood depends on the glucose concentration, only the blood layers are modeled as Cole-Cole materials in (Figure 3.2). The remaining layers in (Figure 3.2) are defined as a homogeneous dielectric material and have a fixed permittivity.

The human finger model consists of skin, fat, bone, blood, and nail layers. The size of the model is 20 mm × 15 mm × 10.5 mm. The nail layer *hf1* (*hf* - *human finger*) *is* shorter than the others - 13 mm.

The thickness, dielectric constant, and dielectric loss tangent of the different layers of the finger model for 2 GHz are given in Table 2.1 [44,45,46,47]:

Table 3.1 - Layers of the human finger model and their thickness

| Layers of the finger model | Thickness (mm) | Dielectric constant | Dielectric loss tangent | Frequency (GHz) |
|---|---|---|---|---|
| hf1 | 0.4 | 3 | 0.25 | 2 |
| hf2 | 1 | 38.53 | 0.3 | |

| hf3 | 0.5 | 5.32 | 0.19 | |
| hf4 | 1.5 | Cole-Cole model | 0.27 | |
| hf5 | 4.1 | 20.86 | 0.14 | |

The change in the dielectric constant of the finger phantom for different values of glucose concentration from 72 to 600 mg/dL is shown in (Table 3.2) [48]:

Table 3.2 - Dielectric constant of blood at different values of glucose level

| Blood glucose concentration (mg/dL) | Dielectric constant of blood for 2 GHz |
| --- | --- |
| 72 | 70.02 |
| 216 | 69.98 |
| 330 | 69.96 |
| 600 | 69.88 |

Figure 3.4 shows the final model of the human finger phantom:

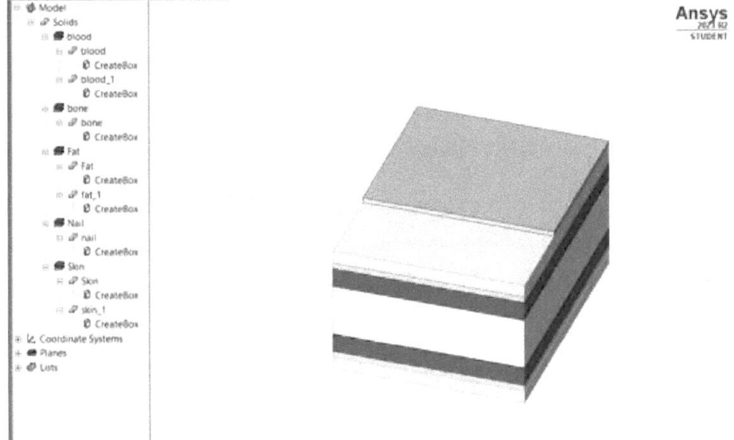


Figure 3.4 - Finger phantom model created in the *Ansys HFSS* software environment

In the *ANSYS HFSS* software environment, it is possible to specify a linear and exponential change in a certain material characteristic with a clearly defined start, end, and step. To model the change in glucose in the material "blood", its dielectric *constant* was set as the parameter "$esp" (Fig.

3.5). Due to the peculiarities of the program, it was impossible to name this parameter by any other name.

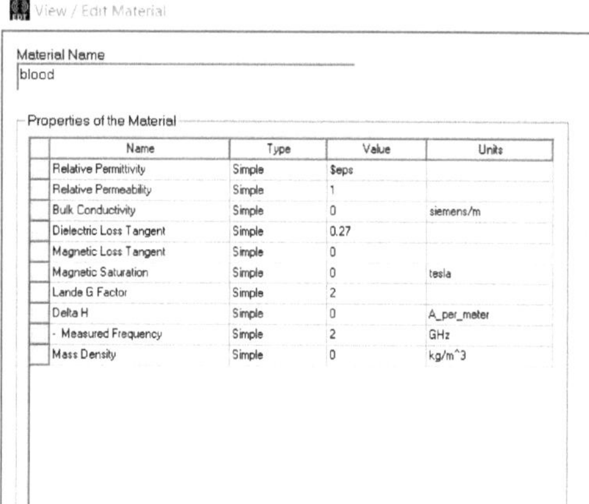

Figure 3.5 - Dielectric constant parameter created in the *Ansys HFSS* software environment

Figure 3.6 shows how the variation of the dielectric constant in the material "blood" was made to analyze the change in glucose.

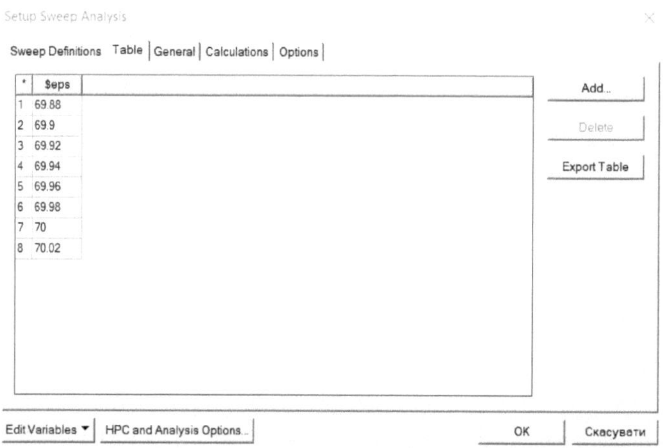

Figure 3.6 - Changes in the dielectric constant in the material "blood" created in the *Ansys HFSS* software environment

## 3.3 Design of a rectangular microstrip antenna

The antenna design is shown in (Fig. 3.7):

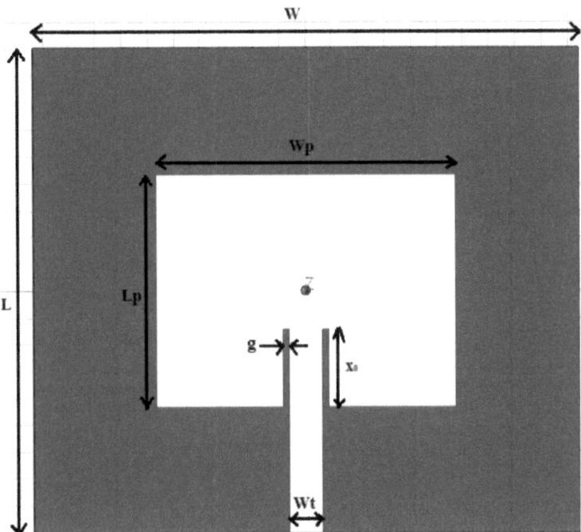


Figure 3.7 - Microstrip antenna design created in the *Ansys HFSS* software
environment

The calculated antenna parameters are given in (Table 3.3):

Table 3.3 - Calculated antenna parameters

| Parameter | Meaning. |
|---|---|
| W | 82.5 |
| L | 72.3 |
| $W_p$ | 45.6 |
| $L_p$ | 35 |
| g | 0.83 |
| $x_0$ | 11.8 |
| $W_t$ | 2.5 |

The following steps were taken to build the antenna model:

1.  Declare a constant

Figure 3.8 shows the variables that were declared as constants. Thanks
to this, it was possible to use them to set the parameters and location of the
patch antenna parts without rewriting the values.

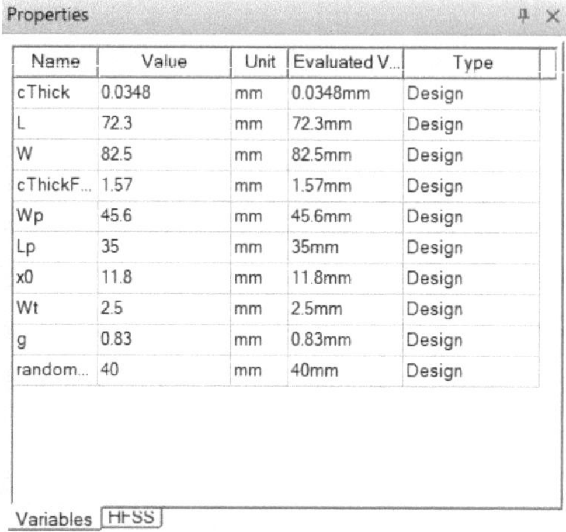

Figure 3.8 - Declaring antenna parameters as constants created in the *Ansys HFSS* software environment

2. Create a metal screen

The metal shield and the radiating element were made of copper with a thickness of *cThick of* 0.0348 mm (Fig. 3.9):

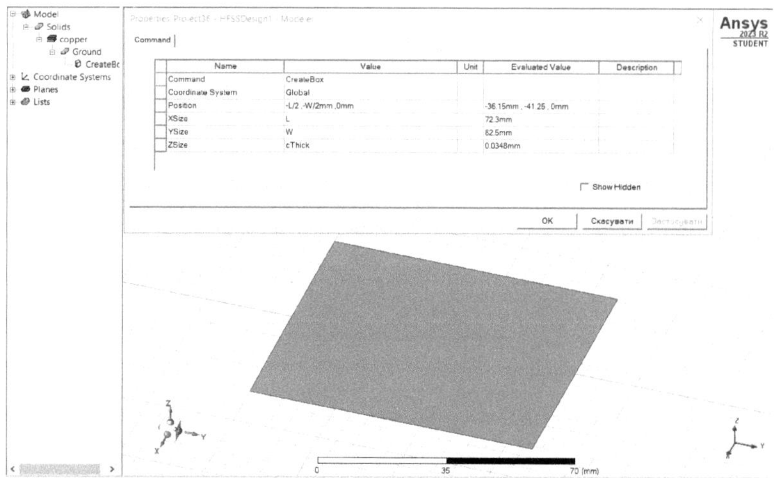

Figure 3.9 - Metal screen created in the *Ansys HFSS* software environment

3. Create a dielectric substrate

The dielectric substrate has the same design parameters as the metal screen, except for the thickness of *cThickFR4* - 1.57 mm (Fig. 3.10):

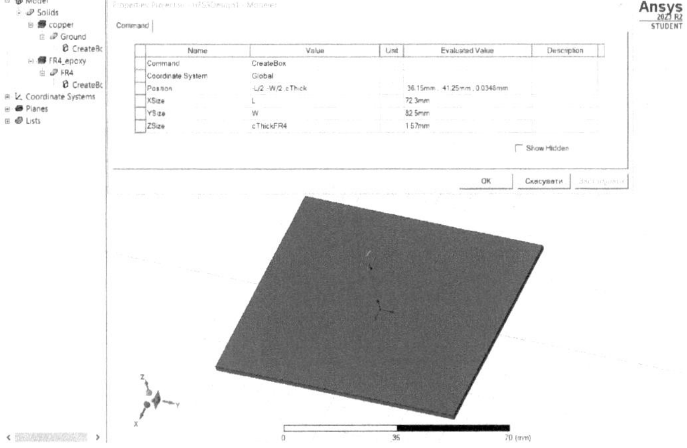

Figure 3.10 - Dielectric substrate created in the *Ansys HFSS* software environment

4. Create a radiating element

A radiating element with a rectangular configuration is shown in (Fig. 3.11).

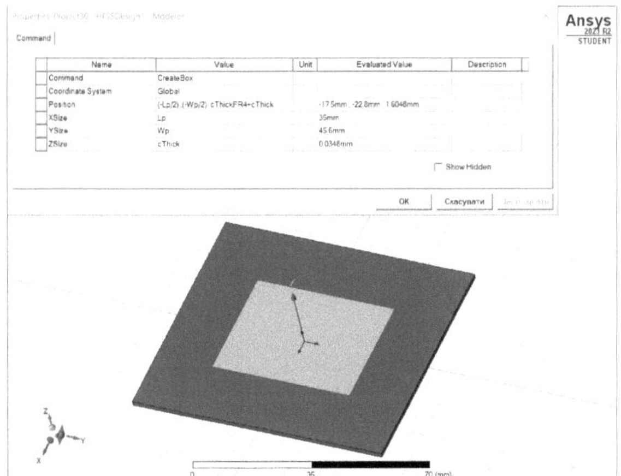

Figure 3.11 - Radiating element with a rectangular configuration created in the *Ansys HFSS* software environment

5. Create a microstrip line

This antenna will be powered by a microstrip line. For the correct connection, you must first build a rectangle - the part that will be "removed" from the radiating element and which is the place of power connection. This list of actions is shown in (Fig. 3.12) and (Fig. 3.13):

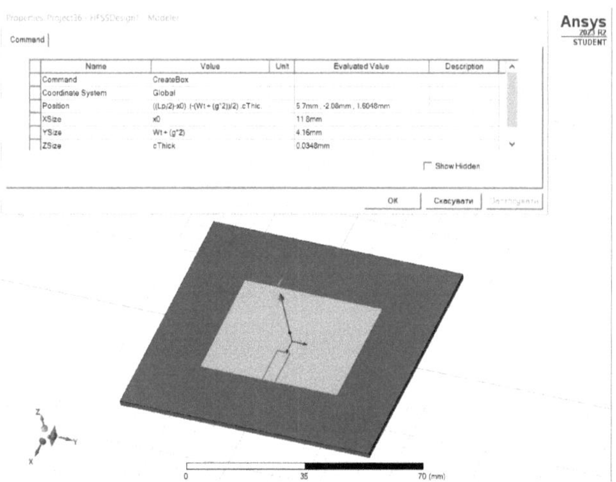

Figure 3.12 - Rectangle at the power supply location created in the *Ansys HFSS* software environment

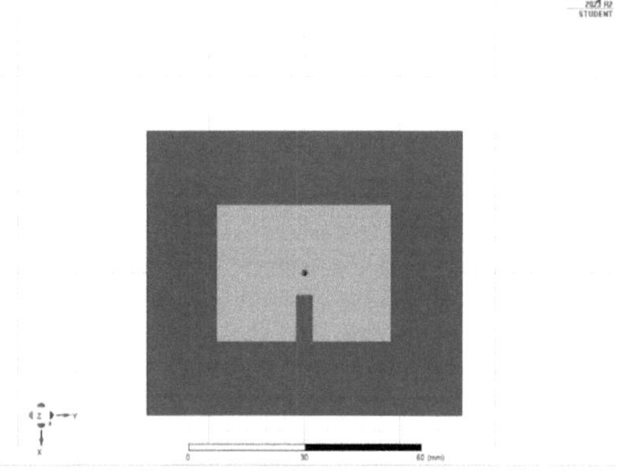

Figure 3.13 - Power connection point created in the *Ansys HFSS* software environment

The next step is to create a microstrip line. Since the shapes will be merged, the *randomhight* parameter can be any distance, as long as it is greater than 30.45 mm and less than 53.65 mm (Figure 3.14). The final result is shown in (Figure 3.14) and (Figure 3.15):

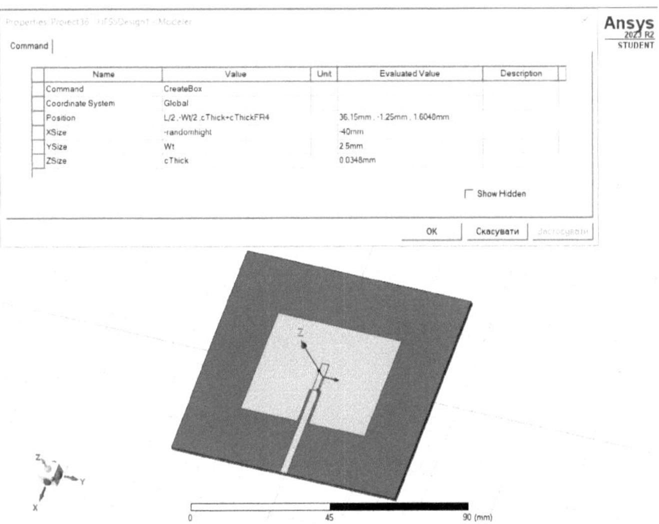

Figure 3.14 - Microstrip line created in the *Ansys HFSS* software environment

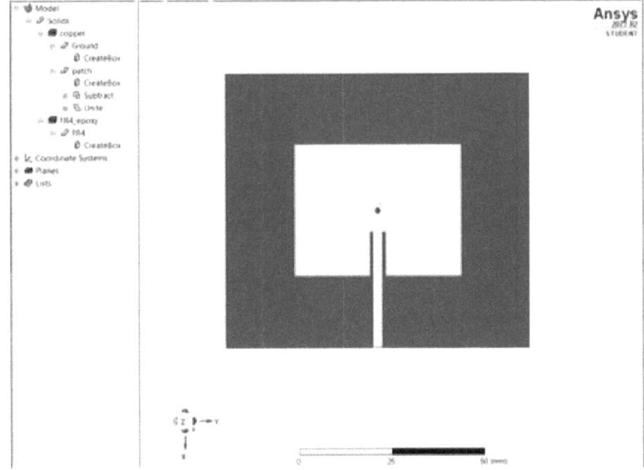

Figure 3.15 - Final result created in the *Ansys HFSS* software
environment

5. Create a Lumped Port

*Lumped Port* is an electromagnetic signal source that is created only
to power a microstrip line. This process is shown in (Figure 3.16) and (Figure
3.17):

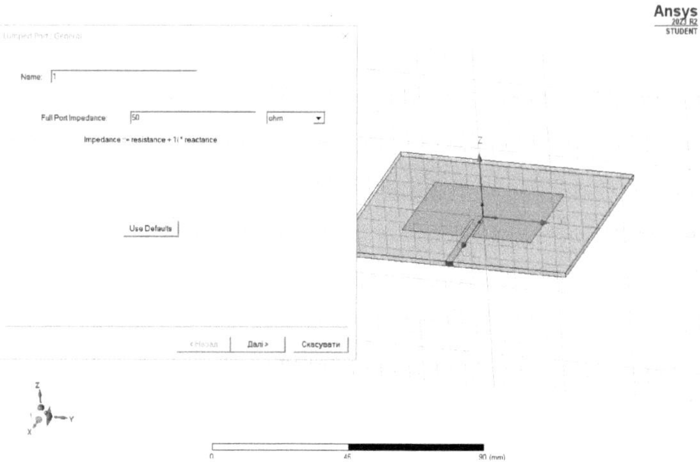

Figure 3.16 - Creating an electromagnetic signal source in the *Ansys*
*HFSS* software environment

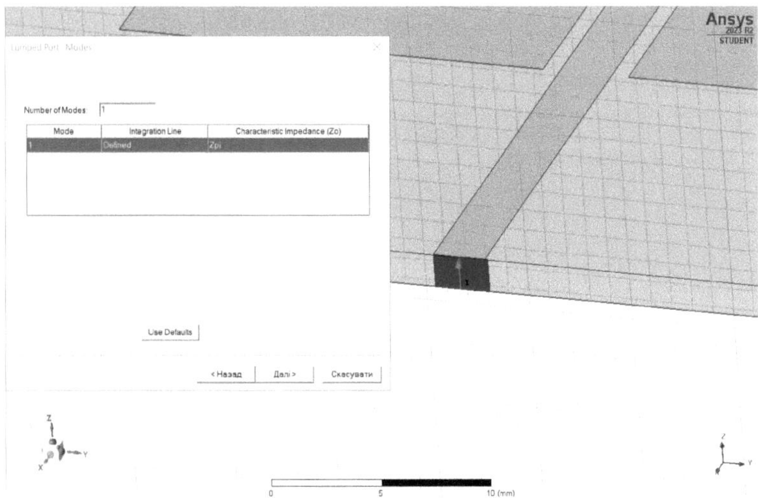

Figure 3.17 - *Lumped port* settings created in the *Ansys HFSS* software environment

6. Create a radiation zone

To model the radiation of the patch antenna and calculate its characteristics, you need to create an *open region* in (Figure 3.18):

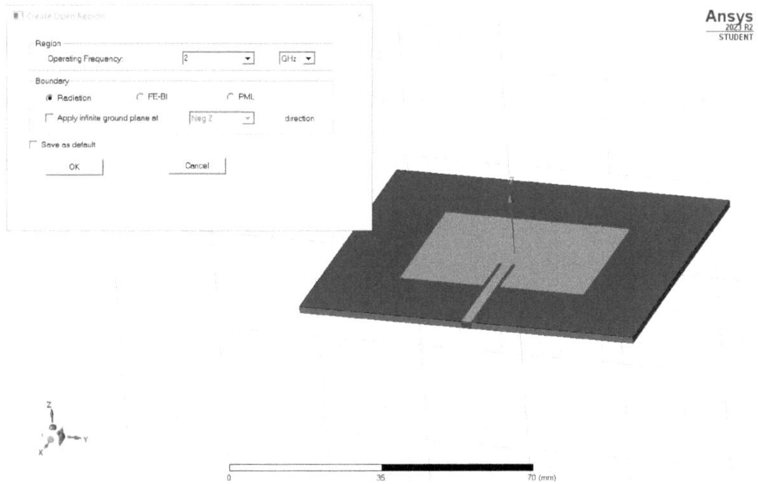

Figure 3.18 - Antenna radiation pattern created in the *Ansys HFSS* software environment

This is the final step in creating a patch antenna.


## 3.4 Modeling results


To investigate the effect of different glucose concentrations in the finger phantom (72, 216, 330, and 600 mg/dL) on the antenna performance, we performed a simulation.

The modeling parameters are shown in **Table 3.4**:

Table 3.4 - Modeling parameters and their values

| Modeling parameters | Meaning. |
|---|---|
| Units of measurement | The parameters of the patch antenna and the phantom finger model are designed in mm. The frequency range of the antenna is defined in GHz |
| Frequency range | 1 - 3 GHz |
| Resonant frequency of the antenna | 2 GHz |
| Source. | Lumped port |

The simulation setup for the resonant frequency of 2 GHz is shown in (Fig. 3.19):

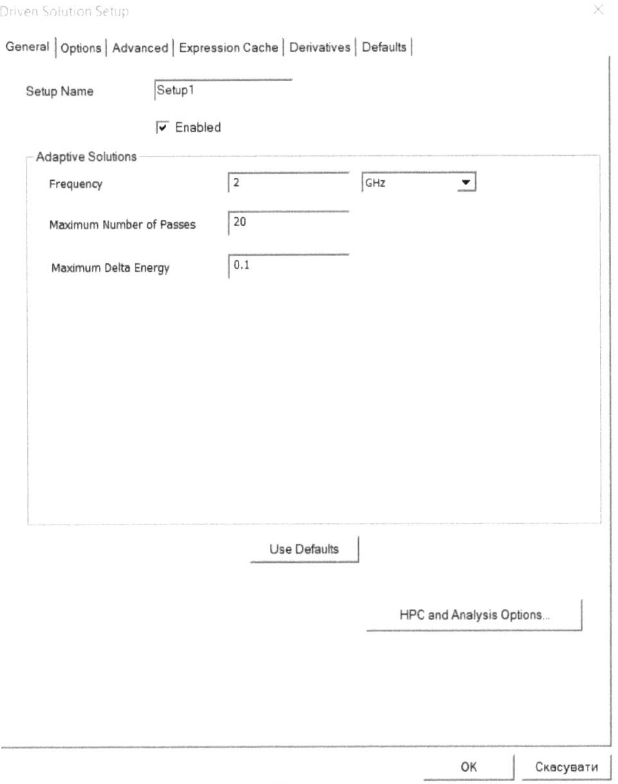

Figure 3.19 - Simulation setup created in the *Ansys HFSS* software environment

### 3.4.1 The result of patch antenna modeling

An antenna's gain is a measure of its ability to radiate the power transmitted by the transmitter in the direction of the target. It is typically expressed in decibels (*dBi)* and is a logarithmic value (3.1):

$$G = 10 \cdot \log_{10}\left(\frac{E}{E_i}\right) \qquad (3.1)$$

where, $E$ *is* the field strength of the antenna at a certain point, $E_i$ - is the field strength of an isotropic antenna at the same point.

The antenna gain (unit *dB)* with a resonant frequency of 2 GHz is shown in (Fig. 3.20):

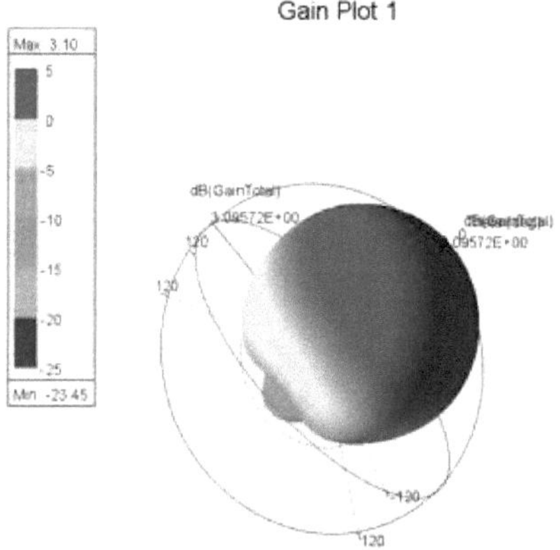


Figure 3.20 - Antenna gain

The E-plane shows the direction of maximum radiation. The *H-plane* contains the magnetic field vector. Figure 3.21 shows the simulated radiation patterns in the *E-* and *H-planes* at 2 GHz.

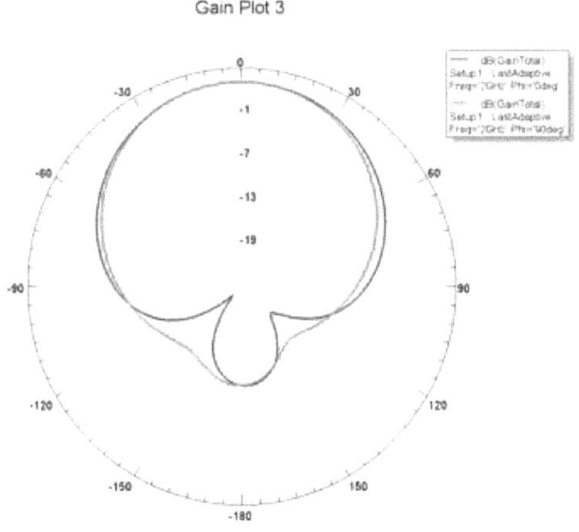


Figure 3.21 - Antenna pattern diagrams

The obtained radiation patterns in (Fig. 3.21) show that the antenna is oriented at an angle of 0 degrees in the E-plane and *H-plane*.

*The S-parameter of the* antenna with a resonant frequency of 2 GHz is shown in (Fig. 3.22):

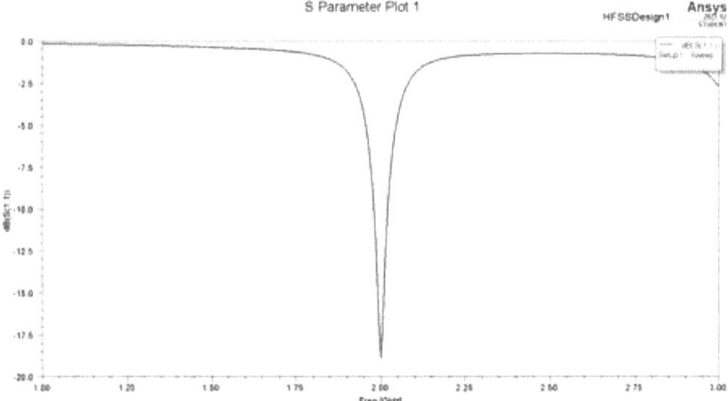


Figure 3.22 - *S-parameter of the* antenna

## 3.4.2 Result of modeling the patch antenna and the phantom finger model

The sensor was located close to the finger model to maximize the interaction of the near field with biological materials (Fig. 3.33):

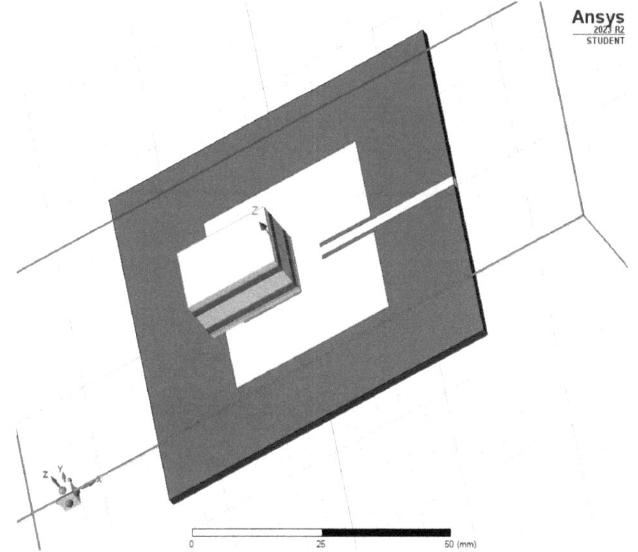


Figure 3.33 - Location of the finger phantom model relative to the antenna created in the *Ansys HFSS* software environment

A comparison of the *return loss* for different glucose concentrations is shown in (Figure 3.34). You can see that the graphs are not easily distinguishable. This is due to small changes in the dielectric constant. When zooming in on a small area at 2 GHz, it can be seen that the most prominent reflected signal is observed for the finger model at $\varepsilon_r = 70.02$ (72 mg/dL) in the blood. As the glucose concentration increases, the dielectric constant of the blood and the *return loss* decreases. The rest of the values differ only by thousandths. Thus, the values for concentrations of 72, 216, 330 and 600 mg/dl are - 6.8195, - 6.8176, - 6.8175 and -6.8171 dB, respectively.

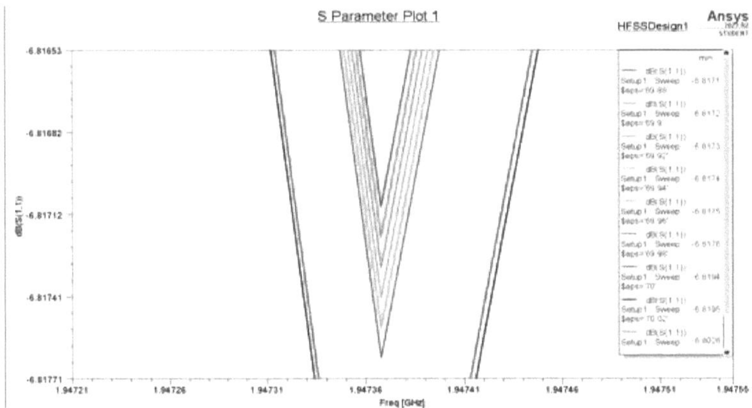

Figure 3.34 - Comparison of *return loss* for different glucose concentrations created in the *Ansys HFSS* software environment

Conclusions to the section III

In this section, we analyze the effect of different concentrations of glucose in the finger phantom on the operation of a rectangular microstrip antenna. Using the *Ansys HFSS* software to model the electromagnetic behavior of antenna structures, it was found that an increase in the concentration of glucose in human blood leads to a decrease in the dielectric constant of tissues, which in turn affects the antenna parameters.

The modeling results showed that at different blood glucose concentrations there are slight changes in the *return loss of the* antenna at 2 GHz. The most noticeable signal is observed with a glucose concentration of 72 mg/dL, which corresponds to the dielectric constant of blood of 70.02.

**SECTION IV**

**LABOR PROTECTION**

**4.1 Characteristics of the device for measuring the level of glucose in human blood**

**4.1.1 Characteristics of the device components**

The main technical characteristics of the device components are given in (Table 4.1) [49]:

Table 4.1 - Technical characteristics of the components of the device for measuring the level of glucose in human blood

| № | Name | Technical characteristics | Quantity. |
|---|---|---|---|
| 1 | Patch antenna | Resonant frequency: 2 GHz<br>Gain: 3.10 dBi<br>Antenna dimensions: 72.3 x 82.5 x 1.6 mm<br>Operating frequency range: 1-3 GHz<br>Input impedance: 50 ohms<br>Dielectric substrate material: *FR4*<br>Radiating element material: copper<br>Return loss: 19 *dB* | 2 |
| 2 | Vector analyzer of electrical circuits *MS2037C* | Operating frequency range: 5 kHz - 15 GHz<br>Spectrum analysis: 9 kHz - 15 GHz<br>RF power meter: 10 MHz - 18 GHz<br>Weight: 4.8 kg<br>Operating temperature: -10°C to +55°C | 1 |
| 3 | Coaxial cable *RG 8 TZC 500 32* | Outer diameter: 10.16 mm<br>Dielectric: polyethylene foam<br>Dielectric diameter: 7.25 mm<br>Screen: aluminum foil (Al)<br>Central core material: copper-plated aluminum<br>Operating temperature: -40°C to +80°C | 2 |
| 4 | *SMA* connector *(female)* | Material: copper<br>Impedance: 50 ohms<br>Maximum frequency: 6 GHz<br>Operating temperature: -40°C to +85°C | 2 |

52

**4.1.2 Components of the device for measuring the level of glucose in human blood**

The functional diagram of the device is shown in (Fig. 4.1):

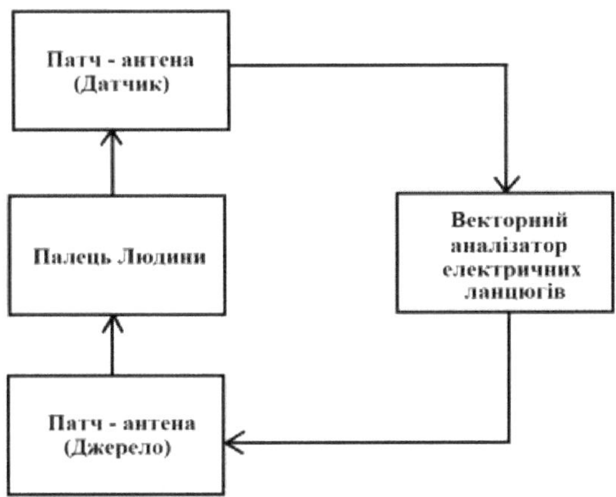


Figure 4.1 - Functional diagram of the device

One patch antenna serves as the transmitting antenna (Source) and the other as the receiving antenna (Sensor). A human finger is placed between these two antennas. The antennas (with *SMA connector) are* connected to the vector circuit analyzer with coaxial cables to record return loss data.

**4.1.3 The nature of the object's interaction in the human-object system**

The means for obtaining information about the patch antenna operation are given in (Table 4.2):

Table 4.2 - Object interaction in the human-object system

| № | Name of the device component | Type of information display | Quantity. |
|---|---|---|---|
| 1 | Display of the MS2037C vector circuit analyzer | Information about the interaction of the patch antenna and the human finger, the analyzer operation | 1 |

## 4.2 Evaluation of potential hazards posed by the design of the device to be designed and measures to eliminate them

### 4.2.1 Risk of electric shock

The source, causes, and consequences of electric shock hazards are shown in Table 4.3:

Table 4.3 - Risk of electric shock

| № | Name of the device component | Source of danger | Causes of danger | Consequences of the danger |
|---|---|---|---|---|
| 1 | Vector analyzer of electrical circuits *MS2037C* | Electrical power supply of the analyzer | Improper use or maintenance of the equipment. Damage to internal components due to overvoltage | Burns on the body, loss of consciousnes s, severe muscle contractions, convulsions |
| 2 | Coaxial cable *RG 8 TZC 500 32* | The electric current that flows through a cable. | Damage to the insulation. Wear and tear of the cable over time | |
| | | Static electricity | Coaxial cables often accumulate static electricity. If you allow a discharge to occur as a result of a direct connection to the | |

| | | | MS2037C analyzer without first discharging the static electricity, the MS2037C analyzer may be damaged. | |
|---|---|---|---|---|
| 3 | *SMA* connector (*female*) | Electric current | Incorrect connection or disconnection under voltage. Damage to the connectors due to mechanical impact or wear. | |

The actual and standard values of the electric shock hazard factor are given in Table 4.4:

Table 4.4 - Real and regulatory hazards

| № | Danger factor | Real value | Normative values |
|---|---|---|---|
| 1 | Direct current | The MS2037C analyzer operates from a 12 V DC source, up to 0.5 A. AC-DC adapters (Anritsu code: *40-168-R, 806-141-R) are* used. | Threshold detectable current: 5.0 - 7.0 mA |

Measures to prevent the risk of electric shock to humans are given in (Table 4.5):

Table 4.5 - Measures to prevent the risk of electric shock to humans

| Group of nomenclature measures for OP | Type of event | Selection criterion |
|---|---|---|
| Technological measures | When using the Anritsu: *806-141-R* adapter, *make sure that the* power supply is at least 60 W at 12 *VDC* | If the power supply is unable to provide the required power (60 W), this may lead to unstable operation of the device |
| | Make sure that the connectors are free of dirt | This helps to ensure electrical contact |
| | Discharge static before connecting coaxial cables to the *MS2037C* analyzer. | Connecting coaxial cables without first discharging the static charge can lead to dangerous electrical discharges, which is |

|  |  | potentially dangerous for both the equipment and the user |
| Operational measures | Comply with all operating rules and regulations. Check cable connections before use. Check cables for mechanical damage before use | Reducing the risk of electric shock to people |
| Organization al measures | Conducting explanatory work on the operation of the device. Users of the device should follow the procedures described in the standards *JEDEC-625 (EIA-625), MIL-HDBK-263*. | The instructions and explanations help to avoid misuse of the appliance, which can lead to personal injury. |

## 4.2.2 Fire hazard

The source, causes, and consequences of fire hazards are shown in Table 4.6:

Table 4.6 - Fire hazard

| № | Name of the device component | Source of danger | Causes of danger | Consequences of the danger |
|---|---|---|---|---|
| 1 | Vector analyzer of electrical circuits *MS2037C* | Leakage current | Incorrect grounding of the vector analyzer | Destruction of equipment. Fire can lead to loss of life |
| 2 | Coaxial cable *RG 8 TZC 500 32* | Electric current flowing through a cable | Overheating of coaxial cables |  |

The actual and standard values of the fire hazard factor are shown in Table 4.7:

Table 4.7 - Real and regulatory hazards

| № | Danger factor | Real value | Normative values |
|---|---|---|---|
| 1 | Temperature of coaxial cable *RG 8 TZC 500 32* | -40°C to +80°C | To avoid damage to the cable insulation, the maximum permissible temperature should not exceed +80°C |
| 2 | Current flowing through a coaxial cable | < 10 A | The maximum permissible current for the *RG 8 TZC* |

| | | | *500 32* coaxial cable is up to 10 A. |

Measures to prevent fire hazards are listed in Table 4.8:

Table 4.8 - Measures to prevent fire hazards

| Group of nomenclature measures for OP | Type of event | Selection criterion |
|---|---|---|
| Technological measures | If the adapter plug becomes hot, stop using the *MS2037C* analyzer. | An overheated plug can cause an ignition, resulting in a fire. |
| | When using an *AC-DC* adapter, always use a three-wire power cord that plugs into a three-pronged outlet. | If you apply power without grounding, there is a risk of overheating of components or wiring, which can cause a fire. |

Continuation of Table 4.8

| Operational measures | Comply with all operating rules and regulations. | Minimizing the risk of fire |
|---|---|---|
| Organizational measures | Conducting explanatory work on the operation of the device | The instructions and explanations help to avoid misuse of the appliance, which could result in injury or fire. |

## 4.2.2 Radiation hazards

The source, causes, and consequences of radiation hazards are shown in Table 4.9:

Table 4.9 - Radiation hazards

| № | Name of the device component | Source of danger | Causes of danger | Consequences of the danger |
|---|---|---|---|---|
| 1 | Patch antenna | High-frequency electromagnetic radiation | Antenna operation at high frequencies. Incorrect radiation | Prolonged exposure can lead to serious consequences, |

| | | | settings. Improper antenna design | such as heating of biological tissues. |
|---|---|---|---|---|

The actual and standard values of the radiation hazard factor are given in Table 4.10:

Table 4.10 - Real and regulatory hazards

| № | Danger factor | Real value | Normative values |
|---|---|---|---|
| 1 | Frequency of electromagnetic radiation of the patch antenna | 2 GHz | 10 MHz -300 GHz. (Depends on the exposure time and maximum permissible energy load) |

Measures to prevent radiation hazards are given in Table 4.11:

Table 4.11 - Measures to prevent radiation hazards

| Group of nomenclature measures for OP | Type of event | Selection criterion |
|---|---|---|
| Technological measures | The antenna must be designed in such a way that it has directional radiation. The patch antenna design meets this requirement | Directional antennas emit electromagnetic waves in one direction, thus minimizing the impact of radiation outside the required area |
| Operational measures | Limiting the operating time at maximum power | Reducing the overall exposure of personnel to radiation |
| Organizational measures | Conducting explanatory work on the operation of the device | The instructions and explanations help to avoid misuse of the appliance, which can lead to personal injury. |

**4.3 Development of "Safety instructions for the operation of a device for non-invasive measurement of glucose in human blood"**

1. Perform all technological, operational, and organizational measures described in this section.

2. Clean the *MS2037C* Vector Circuit Analyzer with a soft, lint-free cloth dampened with water.

3. Clean the connectors and center contacts with a cotton swab dipped in denatured alcohol.

4. Inspect the coaxial cables carefully. They must not have any breaks or tears or be deformed or stretched.

5. To prevent accidental disconnection of the coaxial cables during measurements, make sure that they are properly connected and secured.

6. The appliance must be kept in a safe place and at the proper ambient temperature.

7. In the event of a fire, disconnect the power supply and contact the fire department for assistance.


Conclusion to Section IV


In this section, we have considered the functional diagram of the device for measuring the level of glucose in human blood. This device can be conditionally divided into 4 components: a patch antenna, a *MS2037C* vector circuit analyzer, an *RG 8 TZC 500 32* coaxial cable, and an *SMA connector (female)*.

The hazardous factors were analyzed and general rules were provided to prevent or reduce the impact of these factors on the user. The main hazards that may arise are the risk of electric shock, fire and radiation hazards. Instructions for use of this device have also been prepared.

# CONCLUSIONS

As a result of the literature search, the main types of glucometers and their classification were identified, the method of non-invasive glucose measurement using antenna devices was investigated, and the components of the patch antenna of the future device were analyzed.

To calculate the parameters of the patch antenna, we first determined the penetration depth of electromagnetic waves with frequencies starting from 1 GHz. With a decrease in the resonant frequency, the antenna parameters increase, which is an undesirable characteristic for keeping the size and compactness of the device. The final choice was a frequency of 2 GHz, as it is the maximum frequency for the antenna waves to pass through the blood into the human fingers.

A phantom finger model was created to test the antenna. The project took into account the parameters of blood, fat, skin, bone, and nail to approximate the real average human finger as closely as possible: dielectric constant (to track changes in glucose, this parameter is variable in the blood), dielectric loss tangent, and average thickness. The results showed that changes in glucose level, which in turn affects the dielectric constant, have an impact on the resonant frequency of the designed antenna and can be determined.

# LIST OF REFERENCES

1. HEARTS D. Diagnosis and management of type 2 diabetes mellitus. Copenhagen: WHO Regional Office for Europe; 2023. License: CC BY-NC-SA 3.0 IGO

2. "Fundamentals of diagnostics, treatment and prevention of major diseases of the endocrine system": a textbook for 4th year students of medical faculties in the field of knowledge 22 "Health care", specialties 222 "Medicine", 228 "Pediatrics" / S. M. Kiselev [et al: ZSMU, 2021. - 137 c

3. Mhatre, Pratik J., and Manjusha Joshi. "Design and Verification of Noninvasive Wearable Continuous Blood Glucose Monitoring System for Smartwatches." Progress In Electromagnetics Research M 116 (2023): 155-164. [Electronic Resource]. - URL: https://www.semanticscholar.org/paper/Design-and-Verification-of-Noninvasive-Wearable-for-Mhatre-Joshi/508b790911b2fcca1e1bc0697a161ecb82b65b9e - (date of the application 21.04.2024) - Title from the screen.

4. 1. Rak, S. O. "The non-infectious epidemic of diabetes mellitus." Nursing 3: 42-44. [Electronic resource] - Mode of access to the resource: https://www.researchgate.net/publication/368080036_NEINFEKCIJNA_EPIDEMIA_CUKROVOGO_DIABETU - (accessed 10/29/2023) - Title from the screen

5. Shchehol, I. M. "Diabetes mellitus." SHEI "Ternopil State Medical University named after I. Gorbachevsky of the Ministry of Health of Ukraine (2019). doi: 10.11603/2411-1597.2019.1.9989

6. Karabut, L. V., and O. P. Matviychuk. "Diabetes mellitus as a disease of civilization." (2023).

7. Diseases of the islet apparatus of the pancreas [Electronic resource] - Mode of access to the resource:      https://ipep.com.ua/napryamki-diagnostiki-ta-likuvannya/zahvoryuvannaya-ostrivkovogo-aparatu-pidshlunkovoyi-zalozi/gestaciyniy-diabet - (accessed 29.05.2024) - Title from the screen

8. Tronko, Mykola. "Type 1 diabetes mellitus: etiology, pathogenesis, clinic, diagnosis and treatment." (2021). [Electronic resource] - Access mode to the resource:   http://surl.li/udhlj - (accessed 29.05.2024) - Title from the screen

9. Tronko, M. D., et al. "Type 2 diabetes mellitus: etiology, pathogenesis, clinic, diagnosis and treatment." Practitioner 4 (2021): 35-44.

10. Actual approaches to the treatment of patients with diabetes mellitus: a textbook for students, interns in general medicine, endocrinologists and general practitioners. Dedicated to the 80th anniversary of the birth of Doctor of Medical Sciences, Professor V.M. Khvorostinka / L.V. Zhuravleva, O. M. Kryvonosova - Kharkiv: KhNMU, 2019. - 124 p.

11. Molodanova, L. V., O. E. Makarova, and O. E. Makarova. "Assortment Analysis and Quality Control in the Conduct of Commodity Expertise of Glucose Meters" (2017).

12. Blum, Alyson. "Freestyle libre glucose monitoring system." Clinical Diabetes 36.2 (2018): 203-204. [Electronic Resource]: https://diabetesjournals.org/clinical/article/36/2/203/32874 (date of the application 29.05.2024) - Title from the screen.

13. FreeStyle Libre [Electronic Resource]: https://www.freestyle.abbott/us-en/home.html (date of the application 29.05.2024) - Title from the screen.

14. Accu-Chek Guide [Electronic Resource]:      https://www.accu-chek.com/support/products/guide (date of the application 29.05.2024) - Title from the screen.

15. Akku-Chek [Electronic resource] - Mode of access to the resource: https://accu-chek.com.ua/ (accessed 29.05.2024) - Title from the screen

16. Philis-Tsimikas, Athena, Anna Chang, and Lupe Miller. "Precision,

accuracy, and user acceptance of the OneTouch SelectSimple blood glucose monitoring system." Journal of diabetes science and technology 5.6 (2011): 1602-1609. [Electronic Resource]:

https://www.ncbi.nlm.nih.gov/pmc/articles/PMC3262733/ (date of the application 29.05.2024) - Title from the screen.

17. The Ultimate One-touch Select Glucometer Review: What It Is, How It Works, And How To Use It?

https://medbay.in/onetouch-select-plus-glucometer-review (date of the application 29.05.2024) - Title from the screen.

18. Glucometer Longevita Smart [Electronic resource] - Access mode to the resource: https://longevita.ua/ua/goods/glyukometr-longevita-smart-1764499.html (accessed 29.05.2024) - Title from the screen

19. Ahmadian, Nivad, Annamalai Manickavasagan, and Amanat Ali. "Comparative assessment of blood glucose monitoring techniques: a review." Journal of Medical Engineering & Technology 47.2 (2023): 121-130. [Electronic Resource]: http://surl.li/udhug (date of the application 29.05.2024) - Title from the screen.

20. Di Filippo, Daria, et al. "Non-Invasive Glucose Sensing Technologies and Products: A Comprehensive Review for Researchers and Clinicians." Sensors 23.22 (2023): 9130. [Electronic Resource]: https://www.mdpi.com/1424-8220/23/22/9130 (date of the application 29.05.2024) - Title from the screen.

21. Melnychuk D.O. M 48 Analytical research methods. Spectroscopic methods of analysis: theoretical foundations and methods: a textbook for the training of students of higher educational institutions / D.O.

Melnychuk, S.D. Melnychuk, V.M. Voitsitsky and others: edited by Academician D.O. Melnychuk - K.: CP "Komprint", 2016. 289 p.

22. Jain, Prateek, Ravi Maddila, and Amit M. Joshi. "A precise non-invasive blood glucose measurement system using NIR spectroscopy and Huber's regression model." Optical and Quantum Electronics 51 (2019): 1-15. [URL:

https://www.researchgate.net/publication/330922992_A_precise_non-invasive_blood_glucose_measurement_system_using_NIR_spectroscopy_a nd_Huber's_regression_model - (date of the application 07.05.2023) - Title from the screen.

23. Jain, Prateek, Amit M. Joshi, and Saraju P. Mohanty. "iglu 1.0: An accurate non-invasive near-infrared dual short wavelengths spectroscopy based glucometer for smart healthcare." arXiv preprint arXiv:1911.04471 (2019). Available at: [Electronic Resource]:

https://www.researchgate.net/publication/337208754_iGLU_10_An_ Accurate_Non                                                                 Invasive_Near-Infrared_Dual_Short_Wavelengths_Spectroscopy_based_Glucometer_for_ Smart_Healthcare - (date of the application 07.05.2023) - Title from the screen.

24.        What        is        Raman        Spectroscopy? https://www.horiba.com/int/scientific/technologies/raman-imaging-and-spectroscopy/raman-spectroscopy/ - (date of the application 07.05.2023) - Title from the screen.

25. Li, Nan, et al. "A noninvasive accurate measurement of blood glucose levels with Raman spectroscopy of blood in microvessels." Molecules 24.8 (2019): 1500. [Electronic Resource]:

https://www.researchgate.net/publication/332479170_A_Noninvasiv e_Accurate_Measurement_of_Blood_Glucose_Levels_with_Raman_Spect roscopy_of_Blood_in_Microvessels - (date of the application 07.05.2023) - Title from the screen.

26. Villena Gonzales, Wilbert, Ahmed Toaha Mobashsher, and Amin Abbosh. "The progress of glucose monitoring-A review of invasive to minimally and non-invasive techniques, devices and sensors." Sensors 19.4 (2019): 800. [URL:

https://www.researchgate.net/publication/331171140_The_Progress_ of_Glucose_Monitoring-A_Review_of_Invasive_to_Minimally_and_Non-Invasive_Techniques_Devices_and_Sensors - (date of the application 07.05.2023) - Title from the screen.

27. Davison, Nicholas B., et al. "Recent progress and perspectives on non-invasive glucose sensors." Diabetology 3.1 (2022): 56-71. Available at: [Electronic Resource].

URL:

https://www.researchgate.net/publication/357788864_Recent_Progress_an d_Perspectives_on_Non-Invasive_Glucose_Sensors - (date of the application 07.05.2023) - Title from the screen.

28. Shokrekhodaei, Maryamsadat, and Stella Quinones. "Review of non-invasive glucose sensing techniques: optical, electrical and breath acetone." Sensors 20.5 (2020): 1251. [Electronic Resource]: https://www.researchgate.net/publication/339492619_Review_of_Non-Invasive_Glucose_Sensing_Techniques_Optical_Electrical_and_Breath_A cetone - (date of the application 07.05.2023) - Title from the screen.

29. Di Filippo, Daria, et al. "Non-Invasive Glucose Sensing Technol-ogies and Products: A Comprehensive Review for Researchers and Clini-cians." Sensors 23.22 (2023): 9130. [Electronic Resource]: https://www.mdpi.com/1424-8220/23/22/9130 - (date of the application 07.05.2023) - Title from the screen.

30. Alsunaidi, Bushra, et al. "A review of non-invasive optical systems for continuous blood glucose monitoring." Sensors 21.20 (2021): 6820. [Electronic Resource]:

https://www.researchgate.net/publication/355245631_A_Review_of_Non-Invasive_Optical_Systems_for_Continuous_Blood_Glucose_Monitoring - (date of the application 07.05.2023) - Title from the screen.

31. Wu, Juncen, et al. "A new generation of sensors for non-invasive blood glucose monitoring." American journal of translational research 15.6 (2023): 3825.

[Electronic Resource]:

https://www.ncbi.nlm.nih.gov/pmc/articles/PMC10331674/ - (date of the application 07.05.2023) - Title from the screen.

32. Aldhaheri, Rabah W., et al. "A novel compact highly sensitive non-invasive microwave antenna sensor for blood glucose monitoring." Open Physics 21.1 (2023): 20230107. [Electronic Resource].

https://www.degruyter.com/document/doi/10.1515/phys-2023-0107/html (date of the application 04.05.2024) - Title from the screen.

33. AL-Amoudi, Mohamed Abdulrahman. "Study, design, and simulation for microstrip patch antenna." International Journal of Applied Science and Engineering Review (IJASER) 2.2 (2021): 1-29. [Electronic Resource]. - http://surl.li/udhvs (date of the application 04.05.2024) - Title from the screen.

34. Gupta, Dilip, Ashish Duvey, and Shweta Agrawal. "A Review: Microstrip Antenna" (2019). [Electronic Resource]. - https://www.irjet.net/archives/V6/i7/IRJET-V6I7144.pdf (date of the application 04.05.2024) - Title from the screen.

35. Chen, Zhi Ning, et al. Handbook of antenna technologies. Springer Publishing Company, Incorporated, 2016. doi: 10.1007/978-981-4560-44-3

36. Balanis, Constantine A. Antenna theory: analysis and design. John wiley & sons, 2016. [Electronic Resource]. - https://ia800501.us.archive.org/30/items/AntennaTheoryAnalysisAndDesign3rdEd/Antenna%20Theory%20Analysis%20and%20Design%203rd%20ed.pdf (date of the application 04.05.2024) - Title from the screen.

37. Rana, Md Sohel, et al. "A 2.45 GHz microstrip patch antenna design, simulation, and analysis for wireless applications." Bulletin of Electrical Engineering and Informatics 12.4 (2023): 2173-2184. [Electronic Resource]. - https://www.researchgate.net/publication/379600261_A_review_of_245_GHz_microstrip_patch_antennas_for_wireless_applications (date of the application 04.05.2024) - Title from the screen.

38. Bansal, Aakash, and Richa Gupta. "A review on microstrip patch antenna and feeding techniques." International Journal of Information Technology 12.1 (2020): 149-154. [Available in English]. https://www.researchgate.net/publication/323681936_A_review_on_microstrip_patch_antenna_and_feeding_techniques (date of the application 04.05.2024) - Title from the screen.

39. Azizi, Mohamed Karim, et al. "Terahertz graphene-based reconfigurable patch antenna." Progress In Electromagnetics Research Letters 71 (2017): 69-76. [in Russian].

https://www.researchgate.net/publication/320622806_Terahertz_Graphene-Based_Reconfigurable_Patch_Antenna (date of the application 04.05.2024) - Title from the screen.

40. Understanding the Fundamental Principles of Vector Network Analysis [Electronic Resource]:

https://www.keysight.com/us/en/assets/7018-06841/application-notes/5965-7707.pdf (date of the application 12.05.2024) - Title from the screen.

41. Ansys HFSS [Electronic Resource]: https://www.ansys.com/products/electronics/ansys-hfss (date of the application 27.04.2024) - Title from the screen.

42. Cebedio, Maria Celeste, et al. "Analysis and design of a microwave coplanar sensor for non-invasive blood glucose measurements." IEEE Sensors Journal 20.18 (2020): 10572-10581. [Electronic Resource]: https://ieeexplore.ieee.org/document/9088994 (date of the application 21.04.2024) - Title from the screen.

43. Turgul, Volkan, and Izzet Kale. "Sensitivity of non-invasive RF/microwave glucose sensors and fundamental factors and challenges affecting measurement accuracy." 2018 IEEE International Instrumentation and Measurement Technology Conference (I2MTC). IEEE, 2018. [Electronic Resource]. - https://ieeexplore.ieee.org/document/8409712 (date of the application 21.04.2024)

- Title from the screen.

44. Wollina, Uwe, Martin Berger, and Kerstin Karte. "Calculation of nail plate and nail matrix parameters by 20 MHz ultrasound in healthy volunteers and patients with skin disease." Skin Research and Technology 7.1 (2001): 60-64. [Electronic Resource]: https://pubmed.ncbi.nlm.nih.gov/11301643/ (date of the application 21.04.2024) - Title from the screen.

45. Kallepalli, Akhil, et al. "An ultrasonography-based approach for tissue modelling to inform photo-therapy treatment strategies." Journal of

Biophotonics 15.4 (2022): e202100275. [Electronic Resource]: https://pub-med.ncbi.nlm.nih.gov/35044094/ (date of the application 21.04.2024) - Title from the screen.

46. Megdad, Ayman R., Rabah W. Aldhaheri, and Nebras M. Sobahi. "A noninvasive method for measuring the blood glucose level using a narrow band microstrip antenna." Applied Computational Electromagnetics Society Journal 37.11 (2022): 1118. [Electronic Resource]. - https://journals.riverpublishers.com/index.php/ACES/article/download/182 87/17917?inline=1#rS3.F13 (date of the application 21.04.2024) - Title from the screen.

47. Tissue Frequency Chart [Electronic Resource]. - https://itis.swiss/virtual-population/tissue-properties/database/tissue-frequency-chart/ (date of the application 04.05.2024) - Title from the screen.

48. Yilmaz, Tuba, Robert Foster, and Yang Hao. "Radio-frequency and microwave techniques for non-invasive measurement of blood glucose levels." Diagnostics 9.1(2019):6. [ElectronicResource].-https://www.mdpi.com/2075-4418/9/1/6 (date of the application 04.05.2024) - Title from the screen.

49. Series of portable vector circuit analyzers up to 20 GHz [Electronic resource] - Access mode to the resource: https://www.tehencom.com/Companies/Anritsu/MS20xxC_VNA_Master/ Anritsu_MS2026C_MS2027C_MS2028C_MS2036C_MS2037C_MS2038 C-u.htm - (accessed 29.10.2023) - Title from the screen

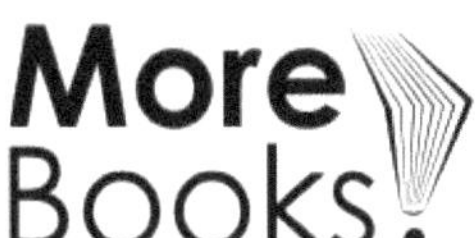

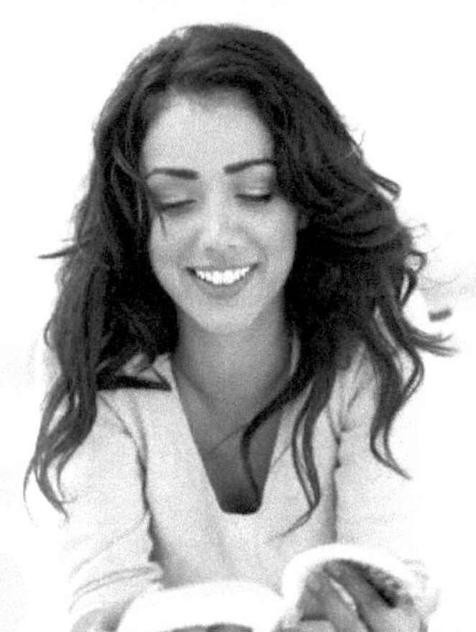

# I want morebooks!

Buy your books fast and straightforward online - at one of world's fastest growing online book stores! Environmentally sound due to Print-on-Demand technologies.

Buy your books online at
## www.morebooks.shop

Kaufen Sie Ihre Bücher schnell und unkompliziert online – auf einer der am schnellsten wachsenden Buchhandelsplattformen weltweit! Dank Print-On-Demand umwelt- und ressourcenschonend produzi ert.

Bücher schneller online kaufen
## www.morebooks.shop

info@omniscriptum.com
www.omniscriptum.com

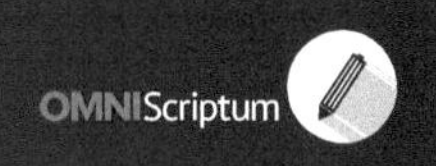

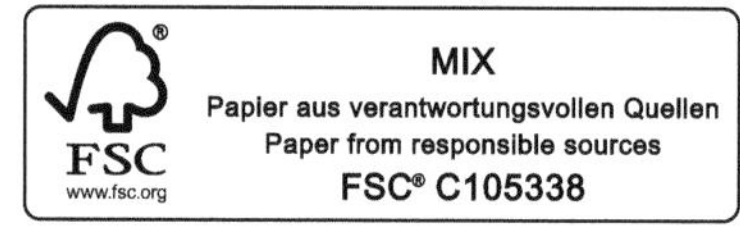

Printed by Books on Demand GmbH, Norderstedt / Germany